T0263325

Enhanced Endoscopic Imaging

Guest Editors

GRACE H. ELTA, MD
KENNETH K. WANG, MD

GASTROINTESTINAL ENDOSCOPY CLINICS OF NORTH AMERICA

www.giendo.theclinics.com

Consulting Editor
CHARLES J. LIGHTDALE, MD

April 2009 • Volume 19 • Number 2

SAUNDERS an imprint of ELSEVIER, Inc.

W.B. SAUNDERS COMPANY
A Division of Elsevier Inc.

1600 John F. Kennedy Blvd. • Suite 1800 • Philadelphia, Pennsylvania 19103-2899

http://www.giendo.theclinics.com

GASTROINTESTINAL ENDOSCOPY CLINICS OF NORTH AMERICA Volume 19, Number 2
April 2009 ISSN 1052-5157, ISBN-13: 978-1-4377-0479-2, ISBN-10: 1-4377-0479-4

Editor: Kerry Holland

Gastrointestinal Endoscopy Clinics of North America (ISSN 1052-5157) is published quarterly by Elsevier Inc., 360 Park Avenue South, New York, NY 10010-1710. Months of issue are January, April, July, and October. Business and Editorial Offices: 1600 John F. Kennedy Blvd., Suite 1800, Philadelphia, PA, 19103-2899. Customer Service Office: 6277 Sea Harbor Drive, Orlando, FL 32887-4800. Periodicals postage paid at New York, NY and additional mailing offices. Subscription prices are $259.00 per year of US individuals $386.00 per year for US institutions, $133.00 per year for US students and residents, $286.00 per year for Canadian individuals, $471.00 per year for Canadian institutions, $362.00 per year for international individuals, $471.00 per year for international institutions, and $185.00 per year for Canadian and foreign students/residents. To receive student/resident rate, orders must be accompanied by name of affiliated institution, date of term, and the *signature* of program/residency coordinator on institution letterhead. Orders will be billed at individual rate until proof of status is received. Foreign air speed delivery is included in all *Clinics* subscription prices. All prices are subject to change without notice. **POSTMASTER:** Send address change to *Gastrointestinal Endoscopy Clinics of North America*, Elsevier Periodicals Customer Service, 11830 Westline Industrial Drive, St. Louis, MO 63146. **Customer Service: 1-800-654-2452 (US). From outside the United States, call 1-314-453-7041. Fax: 1-314-453-5170. E-mail: JournalsCustomerService-usa@elsevier.com (for print support) or JournalsOnline Support-usa@elsevier.com (for online support).**

Reprints. For copies of 100 or more, of articles in this publication, please contact the Commercial Reprints Department, Elsevier Inc., 360 Park Avenue South, New York, NY 10010-1710. Tel. (212) 633-3812; Fax: (212) 482-1935; E-mail: reprints@elsevier.com.

Gastrointestinal Endoscopy Clinics of North America is covered in *Excerpta Medica, MEDLINE/PubMed (Index Medicus), and MEDLINE/MEDLARS.*

Printed and bound by CPI Group (UK) Ltd, Croydon, CR0 4YY
Transferred to Digital Print 2011

Contributors

CONSULTING EDITOR

CHARLES J. LIGHTDALE, MD
Professor, Department of Medicine, Columbia University Medical Center, New York, New York

GUEST EDITORS

GRACE H. ELTA, MD
Professor of Medicine, University of Michigan School of Medicine, Ann Arbor, Michigan

KENNETH K. WANG, MD
Professor of Medicine, Barrett's Esophagus Unit, Division of Gastroenterology and Hepatology, St. Mary's Hospital, Mayo Clinic College of Medicine, Rochester, Minnesota

AUTHORS

HAMZA M. ABDULLA
Medical Student, Barrett's Esophagus Unit, Division of Gastroenterology and Hepatology, St. Mary's Hospital, Mayo Clinic College of Medicine, Rochester, Minnesota

CONSTANTINOS P. ANASTASSIADES, MD
Fellow in Gastroenterology, Division of Gastroenterology, University of Michigan, Ann Arbor, Michigan

LYNN S. BORKENHAGEN, RN
Nurse Practitioner, Barrett's Esophagus Unit, Division of Gastroenterology and Hepatology, St. Mary's Hospital, Mayo Clinic College of Medicine, Rochester, Minnesota

TERESA A. BRENTNALL, MD
Professor, Department of Medicine, University of Washington, Seattle, Washington

MARCIA IRENE CANTO, MD, MHS
Associate Professor of Medicine and Oncology, Division of Gastroenterology and Hepatology, Johns Hopkins University School of Medicine, Baltimore, Maryland

ZHONGPING CHEN, PhD
Professor of Biomedical Engineering, Department of Biomedical Engineering, Beckman Laser Institute, University of California, Irvine, Irvine, California

RAQUEL E. DAVILA, MD
Assistant Professor of Medicine, University of Texas Southwestern Medical Center, VA North Texas Health Care System, Dallas, Texas

JASON A. DOMINITZ, MD, MHS
Associate Professor, Assistant Chief of Academic Affairs, Department of Medicine, Division of Gastroenterology, University of Washington School of Medicine; and Director, Northwest Hepatitis C Resource Center, VA Puget Sound Health Care System, Seattle, Washington

GARY W. FALK, MD, MS
Professor of Medicine, Department of Gastroenterology and Hepatology, Cleveland Clinic Lerner College of Medicine of Case Western Reserve University, Cleveland Clinic, Cleveland, Ohio

ROBERT N. GRAF, PhD
Department of Biomedical Engineering, Duke University, Durham, North Carolina

GERARD ISENBERG, MD
Associate Chief and Associate Professor of Medicine, Division of Gastroenterology and Hepatology, University Hospitals Case Medical Center, Case Western Reserve University School of Medicine, Cleveland, Ohio

RALF KIESSLICH, MD, PhD
Professor of Medicine, Department of I. Med. Klinik und Poliklinik, Johannes Gutenberg University, Mainz, Langenbeckstr, Deutschland, Germany

MENG LI, PhD
Research Fellow, Division of Gastroenterology and Hepatology, Department of Medicine, University of Michigan School of Medicine, Ann Arbor, Michigan

LORI S. LUTZKE, CCRP
Research Coordinator, Barrett's Esophagus Unit, Division of Gastroenterology and Hepatology, St. Mary's Hospital, Mayo Clinic College of Medicine, Rochester, Minnesota

GANAPATHY A. PRASAD, MD
Assistant Professor of Medicine, Barrett's Esophagus Unit, Division of Gastroenterology and Hepatology, St. Mary's Hospital, Mayo Clinic College of Medicine, Rochester, Minnesota

DAVID N. ROBERTS, MD
Digestive Diseases Section, University of Oklahoma, Oklahoma City, Oklahoma

ERIC J. SEIBEL, PhD
Research Associate Professor, Department of Mechanical Engineering, Adjunct Bioengineering, Human Photonics Laboratory, University of Washington, Seattle, Washington

YUTAKA TOMIZAWA, MD
Research Fellow, Barrett's Esophagus Unit, Division of Gastroenterology and Hepatology, St. Mary's Hospital, Mayo Clinic College of Medicine, Rochester, Minnesota

MICHAEL B. WALLACE, MD, MPH
Division of Gastroenterology, Mayo Clinic, Jacksonville, Florida

KENNETH K. WANG, MD
Professor of Medicine, Barrett's Esophagus Unit, Division of Gastroenterology and Hepatology, St. Mary's Hospital, Mayo Clinic College of Medicine, Rochester, Minnesota

THOMAS D. WANG, MD, PhD
Assistant Professor of Medicine, Division of Gastroenterology and Hepatology, Department of Medicine, University of Michigan School of Medicine; and Assistant Professor of Biomedical Engineering, Department of Biomedical Engineering, University of Michigan, Ann Arbor, Michigan

ADAM WAX, PhD
Department of Biomedical Engineering, Duke University, Durham, North Carolina

BRIAN C. WILSON, PhD
Professor of Medical Biophysics, Department of Medical Biophysics, Ontario Cancer Institute/Princess Margaret Hospital, Toronto, Ontario, Canada

LOUIS-MICHEL WONG KEE SONG, MD
Assistant Professor of Medicine, Barrett's Esophagus Unit, Division of Gastroenterology and Hepatology, St. Mary's Hospital, Mayo Clinic College of Medicine, Rochester, Minnesota

JUN ZHANG, PhD
Department of Biomedical Engineering, Beckman Laser Institute, University of California, Irvine, Irvine, California

Contents

Foreword

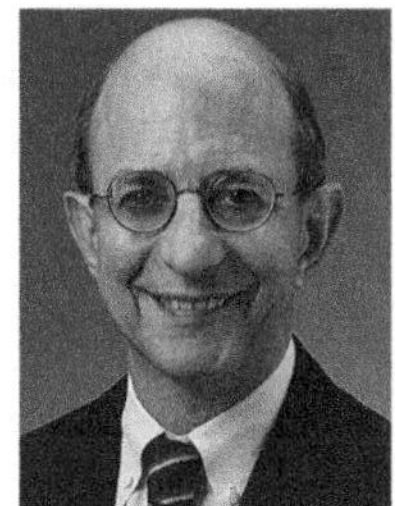

Charles J. Lightdale, MD
Consulting Editor

Not your father's endoscopes, the latest high-resolution scopes have charge-coupled device chips in the tip with more than a million pixels, compared with the standard 300,000. Combine that with a high-definition monitor that scans at 1080 lines compared with the standard 500, and you have a remarkably enhanced image showing detailed views of the gastrointestinal mucosa. But this is only the beginning.

Progress in optical science is now being applied to produce extraordinary gains in endoscopic imaging, never imagined by the fiberoptic pioneers. Some of these new possibilities are already commercially available and are undergoing intensive clinical testing. Others are still in the laboratory phase, but with tremendous promise for the future.

There are two major clinical goals that may require different imaging methods. One is improved detection, which may allow us to find minute abnormalities not otherwise visible even with high-resolution, high-definition systems. For example, it may be possible to detect otherwise invisible premalignant changes in flat mucosa that may be amenable to endoscopic ablation. The second goal is characterization of abnormalities, the "optical biopsy," which could potentially differentiate inflammatory from neoplastic tissue or benign from malignant.

Recognition of the subtle changes and patterns provided by new imaging methods will require considerable training. The question increasingly heard in the endoscopy room is "Do you see what I see?" Until machines can identify, define, and quantify, it will be the human eye and brain that will be the key final step for image interpretation. The potential to improve current endoscopic dilemmas is profound. For example, we might be able to detect dysplastic changes in Barrett's esophagus, replacing random biopsies with targeted biopsies, and greatly improve the detection and diagnosis of flat adenomas in the colon.

Progress in endoscopic imaging is clearly going to benefit from collaborations between endoscopists, scientists, and engineers. I was very pleased when the American Society for Gastrointestinal Endoscopy and the National Institutes of Health combined recently to organize a conference specifically designed to foster this type

Gastrointest Endoscopy Clin N Am 19 (2009) xi–xii
doi:10.1016/j.giec.2009.03.001
giendo.theclinics.com

of cooperation. Sensing that this could be the basis for a *Gastrointestinal Endoscopy Clinics of North America*, I contacted the Directors, Dr. Grace Elta and Dr. Kenneth Wang, widely renowned leaders in gastrointestinal endoscopy, and was gratified when they agreed to be guest editors for this great edition of the *Clinics* devoted to enhanced endoscopic imaging. Every gastrointestinal endoscopist should read these pages to get a clear view of the current state of the art to apply to their current practice and to get a glimpse of the future.

Charles J. Lightdale, MD
Department of Medicine
Columbia University Medical Center
161 Fort Washington Avenue, Room 812
New York, NY 10032, USA

E-mail address:
CJL18@columbia.edu

Preface

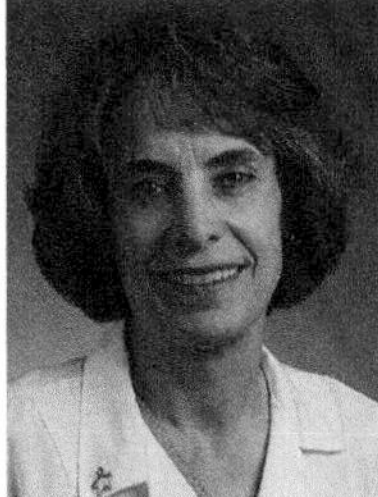
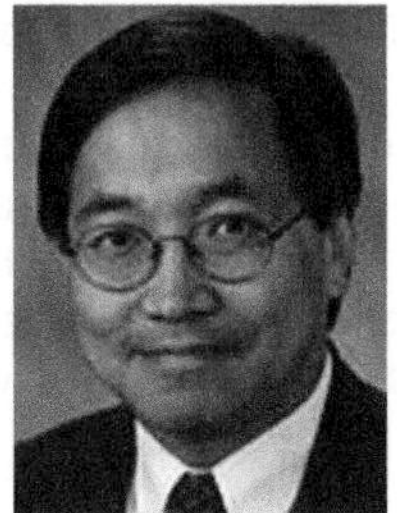

Grace H. Elta, MD Kenneth K. Wang, MD
Guest Editors

Endoscopic imaging is undergoing a profound evolutionary change. Endoscopists have accepted the evolution from fiberoptic imaging to videoendoscopy without enhancements. The next change is the addition of a plethora of imaging modalities that improve visualization of the mucosa. These changes have all been brought about by the need to visualize what formerly was possible only with biopsy and histologic interpretation. Random biopsies, which have been the endoscopic standard, are clearly inefficient and miss significant histology. In addition, flat adenomas and areas of the colon that previously have been difficult to visualize need to be addressed. It is hoped that these new imaging modalities will bring about a new world of endoscopy that can even visualize molecular changes.

The idea for this edition of *Gastrointestinal Endoscopy Clinics of North America* came from a conference organized by the American Society for Gastrointestinal Endoscopy and the National Institutes of Health in April 2007 by Dr. Grace Elta and Dr. Kenneth Wang. It was designed to integrate basic investigators in the field of optics with clinicians who work alongside them. The articles are a reflection of that, with many being authored by scientists and physicians. We hope that the issue will offer insight into the state of the art in endoscopic imaging. The topics included can be roughly separated into two different areas: (1) image-enhanced endoscopy or a red flag technique to survey the entire lumen of the gastrointestinal tract; and (2) virtual histology, which is a "point" technique that can hopefully more specifically diagnose any questionable areas.

IMAGE-ENHANCED ENDOSCOPY

Image-enhanced endoscopy has been classified into two categories: dye-based, or chromoendoscopy, and equipment-based endoscopy. Chromoendoscopy-based techniques include absorptive or vital reactive dyes and contrast stains. The absorptive stains include Lugol's solution, Methylene blue, and crystal violet. Diluted acetic acid is not a dye per se but is a contrast enhancer, because it functions as a mucolytic and alters cellular protein structure. Indigo carmine is perhaps the most commonly

Gastrointest Endoscopy Clin N Am 19 (2009) xiii–xiv
doi:10.1016/j.giec.2009.03.002 giendo.theclinics.com

used dye and is a contrast stain, accentuating borders and surface topography of a lesion by pooling into crevices.

Equipment-based image enhancement includes narrow band imaging and optimal band imaging. These techniques are much simpler and faster to use than chromoendoscopy and may well eventually replace chromoendoscopy. Although there is currently a paucity of comparative trials, the ones that exist suggest that equipment-based image enhancement is as effective as chromoendoscopy. Many experts believe that the major advantage of all image enhancement methods is in the learning curve of how to evaluate subtle mucosal patterns. Once this learning curve has been mastered, careful inspection with high-resolution magnification, white light endoscopy may prove equal in sensitivity.

VIRTUAL HISTOLOGY

Several techniques are under investigation for better inspection of gastrointestinal mucosa with improved detection of dysplasia and early carcinoma. Some of these techniques have not yet shown great promise due to either lack of specificity, such as autofluorescence, or due to lack of improved detection, such as optical coherence tomography. Other methods are still in the infancy of study, such as molecular tagging with subsequent enhanced imaging.

There are two methods becoming established as ways to achieve true "in vivo histology." The first of these is laser confocal microscopy, which is either scope-based or probe-based. The second is endocytoscopy, which has 450 to 1100 times magnification. These technologies require training and interpretation of histology-type images. Although the images achieved with both of these techniques are quite remarkable, it remains unclear how this "on-the-fly" histology will change treatment algorithms. More data and experience are required to sort out the eventual clinical role of these techniques. Spectroscopic techniques that use machine-based algorithms to make the determination of neoplastic probability are also available. These techniques rely on interactions of photons with cellular structures to generate spectrographs of the tissue.

It is unclear at this point which technologies will dominate. One trend on the rise is for mucosal scanning, in which, techniques such as autofluorescence imaging are needed, which are very sensitive and require a point diagnostic technique to establish a firm diagnosis. No single technology will likely achieve all of these goals.

We hope that the reader understands the trends in optical imaging, as discussed in this issue; we also hope that more gastroenterologists are interested in this area.

Grace H. Elta, MD
University of Michigan School of Medicine
3912 Taubman Center
Ann Arbor, MI 48109-0362, USA

Kenneth K. Wang, MD
Mayo Clinic and Foundation
1st Street SW, Alfred M430
Rochester, MN 55905-0001, USA

E-mail addresses:
gelta@med.umich.edu (G.H. Elta)
wang.kenneth@mayo.edu (K.K. Wang)

Chromoendoscopy

Raquel E. Davila, MD

KEYWORDS

- Chromoendoscopy • Dye spraying • Staining
- Barrett's esophagus • Dysplasia • Esophageal cancer
- Gastric cancer • Colorectal polyps

Chromoendoscopy involves the topical application of stains or dyes to the gastrointestinal mucosa during endoscopy to improve tissue visualization, characterization, and diagnosis.[1] Stain or dye solutions are categorized as absorptive (vital), contrast, or reactive. Absorptive stains are taken up by specific epithelial cells of the gastrointestinal tract. Contrast stains are not absorbed, but rather pool in the crevices of the mucosa and accentuate the topography and mucosal irregularities of tissues. Reactive stains respond to the chemical milieu within tissues and undergo a color change based on the presence of an acidic or alkaline pH.

TECHNIQUE AND SPECIFIC STAINS

Stain solutions are generally widely available. Dilution of the staining agents may be necessary, as they are often commercially available in concentrated form. A dedicated spray catheter is usually used through the working channel of the endoscope to deliver a fine mist of the staining solution to the mucosa. Intravenous glucagon or atropine may be used before stain delivery to decrease motility and optimize visualization.

Lugol's Solution

Lugol's solution is an absorptive stain containing iodine, potassium iodide, and distilled water. The solution has an affinity to glycogen in nonkeratinized squamous epithelium, and, therefore, is usually used in the esophagus to detect squamous dysplasia and squamous cell carcinoma.[2,3] Application of a 0.5% to 3% solution to the esophagus results in a green-brown, dark-brown, or black discoloration of the mucosa lasting up to 5 to 8 minutes. Absence of staining results from conditions in which there is depletion of glycogen in squamous cells, such as dysplasia, squamous cell carcinoma, Barrett's epithelium, and inflammation. Intense uptake of the stain can be seen in areas of glycogenic acanthosis.[4]

The free iodine component of the Lugol's solution can cause mucosal irritation, leading to oropharyngeal burning, retrosternal pain, erosive or ulcerative esophagitis, and, rarely, erosive gastritis.[5,6] The topical application of a sodium thiosulfate solution at the end of the endoscopic procedure has been reported to significantly reduce

VA North Texas Health Care System, University of Texas Southwestern Medical Center, 4500 S. Lancaster Road, MC 111B1, Dallas, TX 75216, USA
E-mail address: raquel.davila@utsouthwestern.edu

Gastrointest Endoscopy Clin N Am 19 (2009) 193–208
doi:10.1016/j.giec.2009.02.005 giendo.theclinics.com
1052-5157/09/$ – see front matter. Published by Elsevier Inc.

symptoms after Lugol's staining.[7] Use of the stain should be avoided in patients with iodine sensitivity. Severe allergic reactions have been reported, including bronchospasm in a patient with asthma.[8]

Methylene Blue

Methylene blue is an absorptive stain that is actively taken up by normal, absorbing intestinal epithelial cells of the small intestine and colon. The stain is not taken up by nonabsorptive cells, such as normal gastric or squamous epithelium, but is absorbed by intestinal metaplasia of the esophagus[9] and stomach.[10] Weak or absent staining in the small intestine, colon, or in areas of intestinal metaplasia is indicative of dysplasia, neoplasia, or inflammation. Methylene blue staining has been primarily used in the detection of specialized intestinal metaplasia, dysplasia, and early cancer in Barrett's esophagus. It has also been used in the detection of intestinal metaplasia, dysplasia, and early cancer of the stomach.[10–13]

Chromoendoscopy with methylene blue in the esophagus involves several steps.[14] First, the surface mucus is removed using a mucolytic agent, such as a 10% solution of N-acetylcystein. After approximately 2 minutes, a 0.5% to 1% solution of methylene blue is applied. Staining occurs within 2 to 3 minutes, and excess dye is then vigorously removed with water irrigation. Epithelial uptake of the stain results in a blue discoloration, which is resistant to washing and can persist for up to 24 hours. Excretion of the stain can occur through the urinary tract or by cellular sloughing into the gastrointestinal tract, which can result in greenish or bluish discoloration of the urine and stool.[1,15]

In general, methylene blue is well tolerated, with no significant side effects reported. There have been reports of oxidative DNA damage induced by the combination of methylene blue and white light exposure during chromoendoscopy of Barrett's epithelium and colonic mucosa.[16,17] It has been speculated that this DNA damage can accelerate carcinogenesis in Barrett's epithelium. However, there is no current evidence of increased cancers in patients who have undergone chromoendoscopy with methylene blue in clinical studies.[18]

Toluidine Blue

Toluidine blue or tolonium chloride is a basic dye that stains cell nuclei.[1] It is mostly used in the detection of malignant cells due to their increased mitotic activity and high nuclear to cytoplasmic ratio, which lead to avid stain absorption.[19] Staining of abnormal tissues results in blue discoloration. Toluidine blue chromoendoscopy has been mainly used in the evaluation of squamous dysplasia and squamous cell carcinoma of the oral cavity and esophagus.[20–23] Benign conditions, such as inflammation, erosions, ulcers, and fibrosis, can falsely stain positive.[1,4]

The staining technique involves use of a mucolytic, such as 1% acetic acid, to get rid of surface mucus. Subsequently, a 1% aqueous toluidine blue solution is sprayed topically. After 1 to 2 minutes, a second washing with 1% acetic acid is performed to remove any excess dye.[21] There are no reports of side effects or toxicity associated with toluidine blue use.

Crystal Violet

Crystal violet is a topical antimicrobial agent that irreversibly binds microbial DNA and directly inhibits cell replication.[24] It stains the nuclei of normal and cancerous cells, resulting in a purple discoloration, and is useful for highlighting the surface morphology of cells. Crystal violet staining has been reported to be useful in delineating the pit pattern of Barrett's epithelium[25] as well as polypoid and nonpolypoid lesions of the colon. It has also been used for the detection of early gastric cancer.[26]

The staining process involves using a mucolytic agent before spraying a 0.05% to 0.1% crystal violet solution. Combined use of crystal violet and methylene blue has been described for the detection of dysplasia and early cancer in Barrett's epithelium.[27,28] Furthermore, sequential use of indigo carmine followed by crystal violet has been described for the evaluation of large, flat polypoid lesions of the colon before endoscopic mucosal resection (EMR).[29] There are no reports of side effects or toxicity associated with crystal violet use.

Indigo Carmine

Indigo carmine is a contrast agent that is not absorbed, but rather highlights surface topography by pooling in crevices within the mucosa of a lesion. This in turn helps delineate the lateral extent of a lesion as well as accentuate subtle areas of depression or elevation.[15] Indigo carmine chromoendoscopy has been combined with high-resolution or high-magnification endoscopy to obtain greater mucosal detail and identify surface patterns that can be used to predict histology.[15] The most common use of indigo staining has been in the colon to differentiate neoplastic from nonneoplastic polyps based on the pit pattern; to detect flat or depressed polyps; to evaluate large polyps before and after EMR, and to detect areas of dysplasia in chronic ulcerative colitis (UC). In the esophagus, indigo carmine has been used to detect intestinal metaplasia and dysplasia in Barrett's esophagus.[30,31] In the stomach, indigo carmine has been used either alone or in combination with acetic acid to detect small, subtle cancers and to delineate the margins of flat cancers before endoscopic submucosal dissection.[32,33] In cases of suspected celiac disease or tropical sprue, indigo carmine appears to improve the detection of patchy or limited villous atrophy of the duodenum missed by standard endoscopy.[34]

The staining technique involves spraying a diluted solution (0.1%–0.4%) of indigo carmine directly onto the area of interest. In the colon, topical application of the agent can be focused on a specific lesion, can be limited to a segment of the colon, or may be pancolonic. Furthermore, indigo carmine can be administered orally in an acid-dissolving capsule given 30 minutes before colonic preparation with polyethylene glycol solution.[35] There are no reports of side effects or toxicity associated with indigo carmine use.

Congo Red

Congo red is a reactive agent that changes color from red to dark blue in acidic environments where the pH is less than 3. Acid producing mucosa turns blue within a few minutes, whereas non–acid-producing mucosa remains red. Decreased acid secretion due to gastritis, gastric atrophy, intestinal metaplasia, or cancer leads to the absence of blue staining. Subsequently, Congo red either alone or in conjunction with methylene blue has been used in the stomach for the detection of intestinal metaplasia and early gastric cancers.[36–38] It has also been used to study acid-secreting epithelium in the stomach or in ectopic sites, such as the proximal esophagus and duodenal bulb.[39,40] The stain has been reported to be highly sensitive for the detection of chronic atrophic gastritis.[41] Finally, Congo red has been helpful in determining the adequacy or completeness of vagotomy intraoperatively.[42]

The staining process involves stimulation of acid secretion with pentagastrin (5 μg/kg intramuscularly) 30 minutes before the procedure. Excess surface acid is neutralized with a 0.5% sodium bicarbonate solution delivered topically. A 0.3% to

0.5% Congo red solution is then applied to the area of interest. There are no reports of side effects or toxicity associated with Congo red.

Phenol Red

Phenol red is a reactive agent that changes color from yellow to red in alkaline environments. This method of staining has been primarily used to identify *Helicobacter pylori* in the stomach. The staining process requires topical administration of both urea and phenol red to the surface of the stomach. In the setting of *H pylori* infection, urea is hydrolyzed to carbon dioxide and ammonia, which results in an alkaline pH. The reactive stain then changes color to a deep red in areas where *H pylori* is present. This method has been used to map the distribution of *H pylori* in the stomach and to detect *H pylori* infection in the setting of gastric ulcers, duodenal ulcers, and early gastric cancers.[43–45] Areas of complete intestinal metaplasia do not have adherence of *H pylori* organisms and, therefore, do not stain red.[45] False-positive staining has been reported in the setting of bile reflux.[43]

The staining process with phenol red involves several steps.[45] First, gastric acid secretion is suppressed with either a proton pump inhibitor given orally the day before the procedure or an H_2 blocker administered intravenously 30 minutes before the procedure. Immediately before endoscopy, the patient is given a mucolytic agent, dimethylpolysiloxane 80 mg orally, and an anticholinergic drug, scopolamine butylbromide 20 mg intramuscularly, to reduce gastric motility. During the endoscopy, a 0.1% phenol red solution combined with 5% urea is sprayed over the gastric mucosa. A change in color of the agent is seen within 2 to 3 minutes and can last up to 15 minutes. There are no reports of side effects or toxicity associated with phenol red.

Acetic Acid

The application of acetic acid to gastrointestinal tissues has generally not been considered a form of chromoendoscopy, as the agent does not fall into one of the traditional categories of absorptive, contrast, or reactive stains. However, when used in combination with magnification endoscopy, acetic acid can greatly enhance visualization of surface mucosal detail, vascular pattern, and pit pattern. This combination of acetic acid application and magnification endoscopy is known as enhanced magnification endoscopy (EME).[46]

There are several mechanisms of action of acetic acid on gastrointestinal tissues.[47,48] Normally, during endoscopy, white light reaches the submucosal vascular capillaries through the translucent epithelium. Hemoglobin within the vascular network has a certain absorption spectrum that results in the pink/reddish color of the surface epithelium. Acetic acid causes the epithelial surface to opacify, and this masks the underlying submucosal capillaries, leading to a white appearance of the epithelium. This change from normal pink/reddish mucosa to whitish mucosa is known as the "acetowhite reaction." Acetic acid also results in the depletion of surface mucus by breakage of the disulfide bonds of the glycoproteins that make up the mucus layer. Furthermore, the unbuffered acetic acid comes in contact with surface epithelial cells and causes reversible deacetylation of cellular proteins and a change in the tertiary (spatial) structures of proteins in the nucleus and cytoplasm. In columnar epithelium, acetic acid leads to disruption of the columnar cell-surface barrier, leading to swelling, congestion of the capillaries, and enhancement of the mucosal architecture and pit pattern. These processes are transient, lasting from seconds to a few minutes, and are easily reversible, as the acetic acid is neutralized or diluted.

EME has been primarily used in the evaluation and detection of intestinal metaplasia, dysplasia, and early cancer in Barrett's epithelium.[46,49–53] Acetic acid EME with or without indigo carmine chromoendoscopy has been used in the detection of early gastric cancer and for delineating the lateral margins of broad, flat, and depressed gastric cancers before endoscopic submucosal dissection.[33,54–56] There have also been reports of acetic acid instillation alone or with magnification endoscopy for differentiating hyperplastic from adenomatous polyps in the colon.[57,58] Finally, acetic acid has been used to enhance visualization of neoplastic lesions during screening colonoscopy.[59]

Instillation of acetic acid is performed by using a spray catheter or by directly introducing the solution under low pressure through a syringe attached to the working channel of the endoscope. Approximately 5 to 10 mL of a 1.5% acetic acid solution are delivered to the targeted mucosa. Subsequently, water can be used to remove any excess acetic acid. Normal as well as neoplastic, dysplastic, or metaplastic tissues turn white in the presence of acetic acid. Within seconds to a few (<3) minutes, abnormal tissues develop a reddish color, whereas the normal surrounding mucosa remains white. Eventually, within approximately 3 minutes, normal epithelium returns to its normal color. Given the transient nature of the acetowhite reaction in both normal and abnormal epithelia, repeat instillations of acetic acid may be required.[1] There are no reports of side effects or toxicity associated with acetic acid.

UTILITY OF CHROMOENDOSCOPY IN SEVERAL CLINICAL SETTINGS

Detection of Squamous Cell Cancer of the Esophagus

Lugol's staining is useful in the detection of dysplasia and early squamous cell carcinoma of the esophagus. Most studies using Lugol's have been performed in patients considered to be at high risk for developing squamous cell cancer, including those with head and neck cancer, smokers, and alcohol users.[60–65] In a study of 225 Chinese patients, standard endoscopy had a sensitivity of 62% and specificity of 79% for the detection of high-grade dysplasia and squamous cell cancer.[66] After Lugol's staining, the sensitivity and specificity for high-grade dysplasia and cancer were 96% and 63%, respectively.[66] Overall, Lugol's chromoendoscopy for high-grade dysplasia and cancer has a sensitivity of 91% to 100% and a specificity of 40% to 95%.[66]

Lugol's staining also improves the visualization of the lateral margins of lesions, and this can result in a significant increase in the size of lesions compared with the size estimates obtained by standard endoscopy.[63,66] The finding of multiple, irregular, and multiform areas of absent staining with Lugol's solution is associated with synchronous and metachronous esophageal squamous cell cancers.[67] Finally, Lugol's staining has been used in the detection of local recurrence of metachronous lesions after EMR of squamous cell cancers.[68,69]

Chromoendoscopy using toluidine blue has been used in the detection of dysplasia and squamous cell carcinoma of the esophagus in high-risk populations in limited series.[22,23,70] The combination of toluidine blue and Lugol's staining has been reported to be useful before EMR of early esophageal squamous cell cancers.[71]

Detection of Specialized Intestinal Metaplasia and Dysplasia in Barrett's Esophagus

Methylene blue staining has been the most studied technique for the detection of specialized intestinal metaplasia in Barrett's esophagus; however, there is insufficient evidence to support its routine use for this indication.[15] This is because multiple studies published to date using methylene blue staining with or without magnification endoscopy have shown varying results, with sensitivities of 32% to 98% and specificities of 23% to 100% for the diagnosis of Barrett's esophagus.[72] Several large studies including two randomized, prospective, crossover trials have shown that methylene-blue-targeted biopsies result in a higher detection of intestinal metaplasia compared with random biopsies.[9,14,73–77] However, several smaller studies have shown no improvement in the detection rate using methylene blue, specially in cases of short-segment Barrett's epithelium.[78–82] This large variability in the results may be due to operator experience, differences in technique, and patient populations with different prevalence of Barrett's esophagus.[72] There also appears to be high interobserver variability among examiners in determining the presence of intestinal metaplasia in recorded cases of methylene blue staining.[83]

Some studies have shown that methylene blue staining increases the detection of dysplasia and esophageal adenocarcinoma in Barrett's epithelium compared with random biopsies.[14,74,84] These studies have proposed that areas of dysplasia within Barrett's have decreased or heterogeneous uptake of methylene blue staining.[74] However, several other studies, including two randomized, prospective, crossover trials, showed no improvement in the detection of dysplasia and cancer using methylene blue.[73,79,80,85,86]

There is limited experience using other chromoendoscopy stains in Barrett's esophagus. Lugol's staining has been used to demarcate the squamocolumnar interface and thus improve the detection of Barrett's epithelium in patients with gastroesophageal reflux disease.[8] In a study of 11 patients with known Barrett's epithelium, Lugol's staining had a sensitivity of 89%, specificity of 93%, and accuracy of 91% in the diagnosis of Barrett's epithelium.[87] Crystal violet staining with or without methylene blue staining has been reported to be useful in the detection of Barrett's epithelium, dysplasia, and early cancer.[27,28,88] In a study of 400 patients with endoscopically suspected short-segment Barrett's esophagus, staining with a 0.5% crystal violet solution had a sensitivity of 89.2% and specificity of 85.7% for Barrett's epithelium.[88] The sensitivity and specificity for dysplasia or cancer in Barrett's epithelium were 100% and 66.7%, respectively.[88]

Indigo carmine staining has been used to study the pit pattern of Barrett's epithelium.[8,30,31] In a study of 80 patients with suspected Barrett's epithelium, indigo carmine staining detected 97% of intestinal metaplasia and 100% of high-grade dysplasia and early cancer cases.[30] (**Fig. 1**) EME with acetic acid instillation has been used for the detection of Barrett's epithelium with sensitivities of 77% to 100% and specificities of 15% and 90.2%.[46,51,53,83] However, high interobserver variability has been reported for the identification of intestinal metaplasia.[83,89] Furthermore, there is no current validated or standardized classification system for the pit patterns of intestinal metaplasia and dysplasia identified by EME.[90]

Detection of Helicobacter pylori *Infection, Intestinal Metaplasia, and Cancer of the Stomach*

Phenol red staining has been used to detect *H pylori* in peptic ulcer disease and early gastric cancer.[44,45] When compared with endoscopic biopsy, phenol red has a sensitivity of 92% to 100% and specificity of 84.6% to 95% for detecting *H pylori* infection.[43,45]

Methylene blue staining has been used for the identification of intestinal metaplasia and dysplasia in the stomach. The sensitivity and specificity for the detection of intestinal metaplasia range from 76% to 94% and 87% to 97%, respectively.[10,11,13] Methylene blue staining combined with magnification endoscopy has a sensitivity of 97% and specificity of 81% for the detection of dysplasia.[13]

Staining with Congo red has been reported for the detection of atrophic gastritis, intestinal metaplasia, and gastric cancer.[11,36–38] The combination of Congo red and methylene blue staining has been shown to be useful in the detection of early cancer

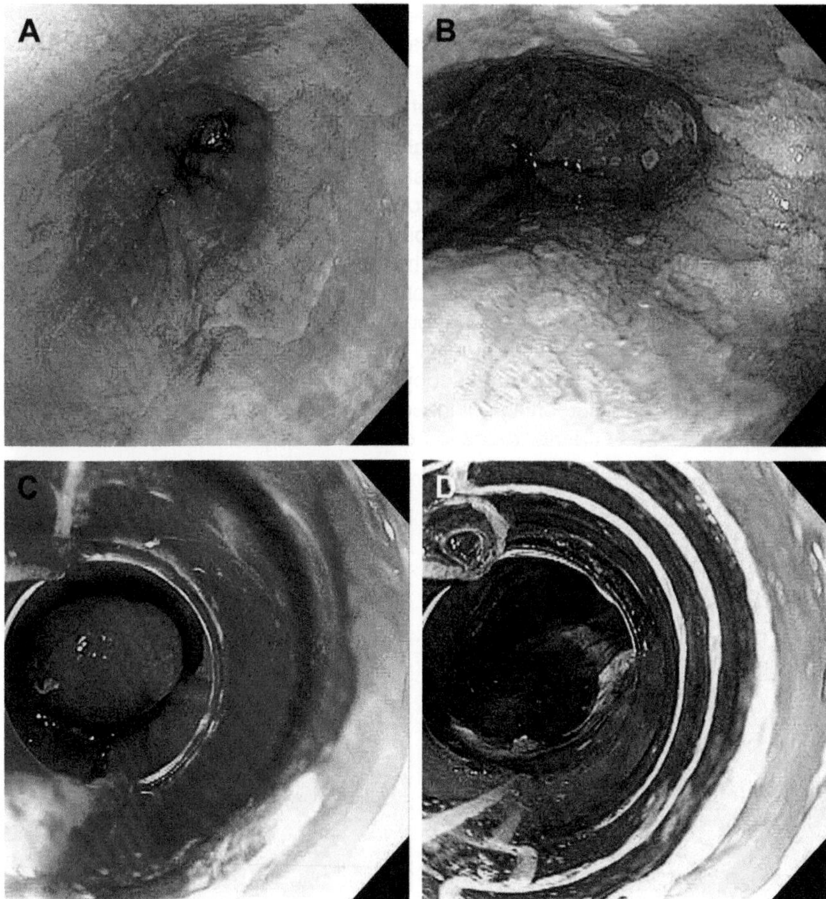

Fig. 1. (*A*) Endoscopic image of long segment Barrett's epithelium with scattered islands of squamous epithelium. (*B*) Chromoendoscopic image with indigo carmine staining showing irregular, villous pit pattern. This was used to direct endoscopic mucosal resection. (*C*) Endoscopic image showing endoscopic mucosal resection of abnormal area using a banding device. (*D*) Endoscopic image of the area after endoscopic mucosal resection. Final histology showed Barrett's epithelium with high grade dysplasia.

and synchronous cancerous lesions missed by standard endoscopy.[37,38] Combined staining of areas of gastric cancer results in pale, bleached areas that do not stain to either Congo red or methylene blue. This combined technique has been used effectively in the surveillance of patients with hereditary, diffuse gastric cancer.[38] Furthermore, the combined test increases the detection of synchronous gastric cancers to 88.9% from the 28.3% identified by standard endoscopy.[37]

EME with acetic acid has been reported for the detection of early gastric cancer. In a study of 45 patients with gastric carcinoma or adenoma, the duration of the acetowhite reaction varied among the different grades of neoplasia, with cancers losing the whitening effect within a few seconds and low-grade neoplastic lesions losing the effect in more than 90 seconds.[54] Subsequently, the duration of the acetowhite reaction may be useful in predicting histology in gastric lesions. Several studies have also reported improvement in the detection of the lateral margins of gastric cancers with acetic acid

EME combined with indigo carmine chromoendoscopy. This, in turn, has been reported to be helpful before endoscopic submucosal dissection of gastric cancers.[33,55,56]

Detection and Differentiation of Colorectal Polyps

Indigo carmine staining with or without high-resolution or high-magnification endoscopy has been used to distinguish neoplastic from nonneoplastic polyps. This differentiation is done based on the Kudo pit pattern classification of colonic lesions in which hyperplastic or nonneoplastic polyps are characterized by round, stellar pits, and adenomatous or neoplastic polyps have tubular, gyrus-like, or irregular pits (**Fig. 2**).[91] In several large studies, the sensitivity and specificity for differentiating adenomatous polyps from nonadenomatous polyps were 82% to 98% and 52% to 95%, respectively.[92–100] All these studies used indigo carmine staining with either magnification or high-resolution endoscopy. In a prospective, randomized study of 660 patients undergoing screening colonoscopy with indigo carmine staining, magnifying colonoscopy was superior to standard colonoscopy for distinguishing between

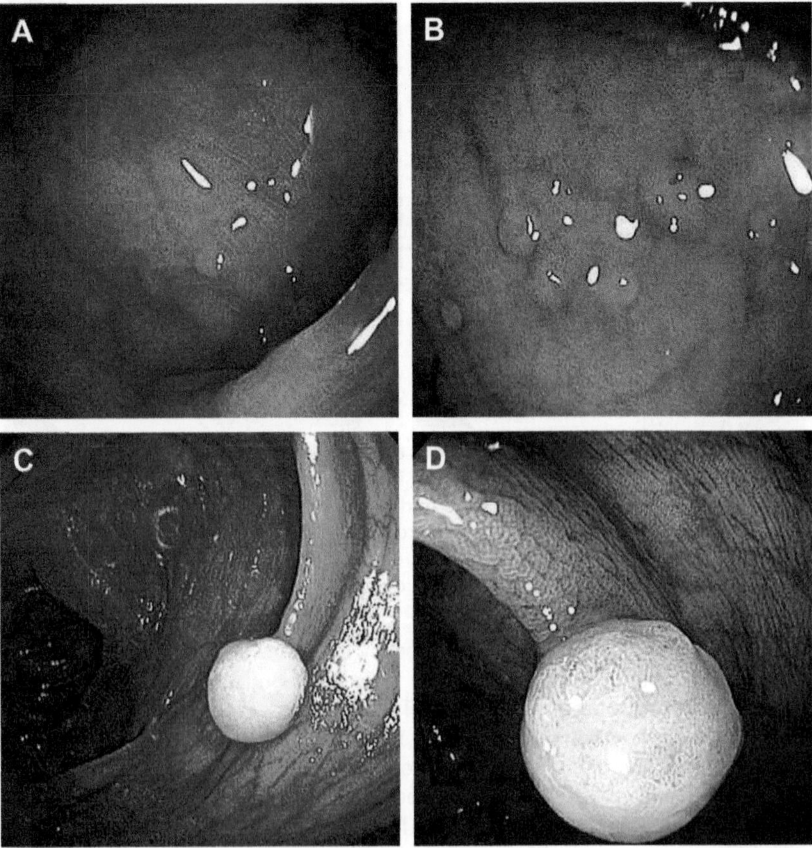

Fig. 2. (*A*) Endoscopic image of several diminutive polyps in the sigmoid colon. (*B*) Endoscopic image of the same area with indigo carmine chromoendoscopy using a standard colonoscope shows several small polyps with rounded pits. Histology was consistent with hyperplastic polyps. (*C*) Endoscopic image of a sessile polyp in the transverse colon. (*D*) Endoscopic image of the same polyp with indigo carmine chromoendoscopy using a standard colonoscope shows a tubular pit pattern. Histology was consistent with a tubular adenoma.

neoplastic and nonneoplastic polyps.[97] The addition of magnifying colonoscopy to indigo staining increased the sensitivity and specificity to 93% and 85% respectively, from 71% and 60% seen with standard colonoscopy.[97] In another study, 150 patients undergoing screening colonoscopy with high-resolution colonoscopes were evaluated for small, less than 5 mm polyps in the rectum and sigmoid colon.[101] The addition of indigo carmine staining to high-resolution colonoscopy only marginally improved the accuracy of distinguishing hyperplastic polyps from adenomas.[101] Overall, the interobserver agreement for determining polyp histology based on pit pattern seems to be good among experienced endoscopists.[102] However, indigo staining with magnification or high-resolution endoscopy has not replaced actual histology in determining a diagnosis of colonic polyps.[1]

Indigo carmine chromoendoscopy has also been useful in the detection of small, flat, depressed, or nonpolypoid colonic lesions.[103–105] In a randomized, controlled trial of pancolonic indigo carmine chromoendoscopy versus standard colonoscopy, there was a significant increase in the detection of nonneoplastic polyps and diminutive adenomas less than 5 mm as well as an increased number of patients with more than three adenomas in the chromoendoscopy group.[106] The withdrawal time was significantly higher in the chromoendoscopy group compared with that in the control group.[106] In another randomized, controlled trial, indigo carmine chromoendoscopy with high-resolution and magnification colonoscopy was compared with standard colonoscopy.[107] Although there was a significantly higher number of hyperplastic polyps and flat adenomas per patient in the high-resolution chromoendoscopy group, there was no significant difference in the total number of adenomas per patient.[107] Finally, in another randomized trial, pancolonic indigo carmine staining was compared with targeted staining directed at specific areas of the colon where there was a lesion in question.[108] There was a significant increase in the total number of adenomas, diminutive adenomas less than 4 mm, flat polyps (hyperplastic and adenomatous) in the right colon, and hyperplastic polyps in the left colon detected in the pancolonic chromoendoscopy group. Despite findings from these three randomized, controlled trials suggesting an increase in the detection of flat adenomas and possibly total number of adenomas per patient, pancolonic chromoendoscopy with indigo carmine has not been widely adopted in routine clinical practice.

Indigo carmine staining with either high-resolution or high-magnification endoscopy has been used in patients with high risk for developing colorectal cancer.[109,110] In two back-to-back studies of patients with hereditary nonpolyposis colorectal cancer syndrome, chromoendoscopy with indigo carmine increased the detection of adenomas, including flat adenomatous lesions.[109,110]

Combined chromoendoscopy with indigo carmine and crystal violet has been used to evaluate flat, broad, lateral spreading polyps before EMR.[29,111,112] Additional chromoendoscopy with indigo carmine has been described immediately after EMR of large, flat lesions to assess the completeness of resection and to rule out any remnant polypoid tissue that would require further removal or ablation with argon plasma coagulation.[112,113]

Detection of Dysplasia in Chronic Ulcerative Colitis

Chromoendoscopy with indigo carmine and methylene blue appears to be useful in the detection of dysplasia in patients with chronic UC undergoing surveillance colonoscopy.[114–119] In a study from Germany, 165 patients with longstanding UC were randomized to standard surveillance colonoscopy versus magnification colonoscopy with methylene blue staining.[114] All patients underwent standard surveillance biopsies every 10 cm and targeted biopsies of visually abnormal areas. In the chromoendoscopy group, there was significantly higher correlation between the endoscopic and the histologic assessment of disease activity and extent. Furthermore, chromoendoscopy had a significantly higher detection rate of flat neoplasia compared with that of standard colonoscopy. Although there was a slightly longer average withdrawal time in the chromoendoscopy group, this difference was not statistically significant.

In a study from Japan, 117 patients with pancolitis for more than 5 years underwent colonoscopy with high-resolution colonoscopes.[116] Standard surveillance biopsies were obtained every 10 cm, and the colonic mucosa was examined first with high-resolution endoscopy and, subsequently, with indigo carmine staining. The sensitivity and specificity for the detection of low- and high-grade dysplasia were 85.7% and 88.5%, respectively, with indigo carmine staining compared with 38.1% and 90.6% with high-resolution endoscopy alone. In another study, 100 patients underwent back-to-back colonoscopies with standard surveillance colonoscopy followed by a second colonoscopy with pancolonic indigo carmine staining.[117] There was a trend toward increased dysplasia detection after indigo carmine staining; however, this was not statistically significant. There was no difference in median withdrawal times between the first and second colonoscopies.

SUMMARY

Chromoendoscopy is feasible and safe for the detection, visualization, and characterization of tissues in endoscopy. Several limitations have prevented the widespread use of chromoendoscopy, including lack of training, lack of standardized classification systems for chromoendoscopic findings, poor reproducibility, unknown cost effectiveness and ultimate impact on patient care, and unknown efficacy compared with newer enhanced imaging techniques.[1] Further studies are needed to address these issues before recommending routine performance of chromoendoscopy in clinical practice.

REFERENCES

1. ASGE Technology Committee, Wong Kee Song LM, Adler DG, et al. Chromoendoscopy. Gastrointest Endosc 2007;66:639–49.
2. Freitag CP, Barros SG, Kruel CD, et al. Esophageal dysplasias are detected by endoscopy with Lugol in patients at risk for squamous cell carcinoma in southern Brazil. Dis Esophagus 1999;12:191–5.
3. Misumi A, Harada K, Murakami A, et al. Early diagnosis of esophageal cancer. Analysis of 11 cases of esophageal mucosal cancer. Ann Surg 1989;210:732–9.
4. Weinstein WM. Vital staining of esophageal and gastric mucosa: not vital but may be helpful. Gastrointest Endosc 1992;38:723–4.
5. Thuler FP, de Paulo GA, Ferrari AP. Chemical esophagitis after chromoendoscopy with Lugol's solution for esophageal cancer: case report. Gastrointest Endosc 2004;59:925–6.
6. Sreedharan A, Rembacken BJ. Acute toxic gastric mucosal damage induced by Lugol's iodine spray during chromoendoscopy. Gut 2005;54:886–7.
7. Kondo H, Fukuda H, Ono H, et al. Sodium thiosulfate solution spray for relief of irritation caused by Lugol's stain in chromoendoscopy. Gastrointest Endosc 2001;53:199–202.
8. Stevens PD, Lightdale CJ, Green PH, et al. Combined magnification endoscopy with chromoendoscopy for the evaluation of Barrett's esophagus. Gastrointest Endosc 1994;40:747–9.

9. Canto MI, Setrakian S, Petras RE, et al. Methylene blue selectively stains intestinal metaplasia in Barrett's esophagus. Gastrointest Endosc 1996;44:1–7.
10. Fennerty MB, Sampliner RE, McGee DL, et al. Intestinal metaplasia of the stomach: identification by a selective mucosal staining technique. Gastrointest Endosc 1992;38:696–8.
11. Tatsuta M, Iishi H, Ichii M, et al. Chromoendoscopic observations on extension and development of fundal gastritis and intestinal metaplasia. Gastroenterology 1985;88(1 Pt 1):70–4.
12. Morales TG, Bhattacharyya A, Camargo E, et al. Methylene blue staining for intestinal metaplasia of the gastric cardia with follow-up for dysplasia. Gastrointest Endosc 1998;48:26–31.
13. Dinis-Ribeiro M, da Costa-Pereira A, Lopes C, et al. Magnification chromoendoscopy for the diagnosis of gastric intestinal metaplasia and dysplasia. Gastrointest Endosc 2003;57:498–504.
14. Canto MI, Setrakian S, Willis J, et al. Methylene blue-directed biopsies improve detection of intestinal metaplasia and dysplasia in Barrett's esophagus. Gastrointest Endosc 2000;51:560–8.
15. Kaltenbach T, Sano Y, Friedland S, et al. American Gastroenterological Association (AGA) Institute technology assessment on image-enhanced endoscopy. Gastroenterol 2008;134:327–40.
16. Olliver JR, Wild CP, Sahay P, et al. Chromoendoscopy with methylene blue and associated DNA damage in Barrett's oesophagus. Lancet 2003;362:373–4.
17. Davies J, Burke D, Olliver JR, et al. Methylene blue but not indigo carmine causes DNA damage to colonocytes in vitro and in vivo at concentrations used in clinical chromoendoscopy. Gut 2007;56:155–6.
18. Dinis-Ribeiro M, Moreira-Dias L. There is no clinical evidence of consequences after methylene blue chromoendoscopy. Gastrointest Endosc 2008;67:1209.
19. Herlin P, Marnay J, Jacob JH, et al. A study of the mechanism of the toluidine blue dye test. Endoscopy 1983;15:4–7.
20. Zhang L, Williams M, Poh CF, et al. Toluidine blue staining identifies high-risk primary oral premalignant lesions with poor outcome. Cancer Res 2005;65:8017–21.
21. Epstein JB, Feldman R, Dolor RJ, et al. The utility of tolonium chloride rinse in the diagnosis of recurrent or second primary cancers in patients with prior upper aerodigestive tract cancer. Head Neck 2003;25:911–21.
22. Seitz JF, Monges G, Navarro P, et al. Endoscopic detection of dysplasia and subclinical cancer of the esophagus: results of a prospective study using toluidine blue vital staining in 100 patients with alcoholism and smoking. Gastroenterol Clin Biol 1990;14:15–21.
23. Contini S, Consigli GF, Di Lecce F, et al. Vital staining of oesophagus in patients with head and neck cancer: still a worthwhile procedure. Ital J Gastroenterol 1991;23:5–8.
24. Wakelin LP, Adams A, Hunter C, et al. Interaction of crystal violet with nucleic acids. Biochemistry 1981;20:5779–87.
25. Yuki T, Amano Y, Kushiyama Y, et al. Evaluation of modified crystal violet chromoendoscopy procedure using new mucosal pit pattern classification for detection of Barrett's dysplastic lesions. Dig Liver Dis 2006;38:296–300.
26. Furuta Y, Kobori O, Shimazu H, et al. A new in vivo staining method, crystal violet staining, for fiberoptic magnified observation of carcinoma of the gastric mucosa. Gastroenterol Jpn 1985;20:120–4.
27. Amano Y, Komazawa Y, Ishimura N, et al. Two cases of superficial cancer in Barrett's esophagus detected by chromoendoscopy with crystal violet. Gastrointest Endosc 2004;59:143–6.

28. Tabuchi M, Sueoka N, Fujimori T. Videoendoscopy with vital double dye staining (crystal violet and methylene blue) for detection of a minute focus of early stage adenocarcinoma in Barrett's esophagus: a case report. Gastrointest Endosc 2001;54:385–8.
29. Hurlstone DP, Sanders DS, Cross SS, et al. Colonoscopic resection of lateral spreading tumours: a prospective analysis of endoscopic mucosal resection. Gut 2004;53:1334–9.
30. Sharma P, Weston AP, Topalovski, et al. Magnification chromoendoscopy for the detection of intestinal metaplasia and dysplasia in Barrett's oesophagus. Gut 2003;52:24–7.
31. Kara MA, Peters FP, Rosmolen WD, et al. High-resolution endoscopy plus chromoendoscopy or narrow-band imaging in Barrett's esophagus: a prospective randomized crossover study. Endoscopy 2005;37:929–36.
32. Ida K, Hashimoto Y, Takeda S, et al. Endoscopic diagnosis of gastric cancer with dye scattering. Am J Gastroenterol 1975;63:316–20.
33. Sakai Y, Eto R, Kasannuki J, et al. Chromoendoscopy with indigo carmine dye added to acetic acid in the diagnosis of gastric neoplasia: a prospective comparative study. Gastrointest Endosc 2008;68:635–41.
34. Siegel LM, Stevens PD, Lightdale CJ, et al. Combined magnification endoscopy with chromoendoscopy in the evaluation of patients with suspected malabsorption. Gastrointest Endosc 1997;46:226–30.
35. Fennerty MB. Tissue staining. Gastrointest Endosc Clin N Am 1994;4:297–311.
36. Asaka M, Sugiyama T, Nobuta A, et al. Atrophic gastritis and intestinal metaplasia in Japan: results of a large multicenter study. Helicobacter 2001;6:294–9.
37. Iishi H, Tatsuta M, Okuda S. Diagnosis of simultaneous multiple gastric cancers by the endoscopic Congo red-methylene blue test. Endoscopy 1988;20:78–82.
38. Shaw D, Blair V, Framp A, et al. Chromoendoscopic surveillance in hereditary diffuse gastric cancer; an alternative to prophylactic gastrectomy? Gut 2005;54:461–8.
39. Nakajima H, Munakata A, Sasaki Y, et al. pH profile of esophagus in patients with inlet patch or heterotopic gastric mucosa after tetragastrin stimulation. An endoscopic approach. Dig Dis Sci 1993;38:1915–9.
40. Mann NS, Mann SK, Rachut E. Heterotopic gastric tissue in the duodenal bulb. J Clin Gastroenterol 2000;30:303–6.
41. Toth E, Sjolund K, Thorsson O, et al. Evaluation of gastric acid secretion at endoscopy with modified Congo red test. Gastrointest Endosc 2002;56:254–9.
42. Schneider TA, Andrus CH. The endoscopic Congo red test during proximal gastric vagotomy; an essential procedure. Surg Endosc 1992;6:16–7.
43. Kohli Y, Kato T, Ito S. Helicobacter pylori and chronic atrophic gastritis. J Gastroenterol 1994;29(Suppl 7):105–9.
44. Tsuji H, Kohli Y, Fujumitsu S, et al. Helicobacter pylori-negative gastric and duodenal ulcers. J Gastroenterol 1999;34:455–60.
45. Iseki K, Tatsuta M, Iishi H, et al. Helicobacter pylori infection in patients with early gastric cancer by the endoscopic phenol red test. Gut 1998;42:20–3.
46. Gelrud M, Herrera I, Essenfeld H, et al. Enhanced magnification endoscopy: a new technique to identify specialized intestinal metaplasia in Barrett's esophagus. Gastrointest Endosc 2001;53:559–65.
47. Lambert R, Rey JF, Sankaranarayanan R. Endoscopy 2003;35:437–45.
48. Canto MI. Acetic-acid chromoendoscopy for Barrett's esophagus: the "pros". Gastrointest Endosc 2006;64:13–6.
49. Gelrud M, Herrera I. Acetic acid improves identification of remnant islands of Barrett's epithelium after endoscopic therapy. Gastrointest Endosc 1998;47:512–5.

50. Rey JF, Inoue H, Gelrud M. Magnification endoscopy with acetic acid for Barrett's esophagus. Endoscopy 2005;37:583–6.
51. Toyoda H, Rubio C, Befrits R, et al. Detection of intestinal metaplasia in distal esophagus and esophagogastric junction by enhanced-magnification endoscopy. Gastrointest Endosc 2004;59:15–21.
52. Fortun PJ, Anagnostopoulos GK, Kaye P, et al. Acetic acid-enhanced magnification endoscopy in the diagnosis of specialized intestinal metaplasia, dysplasia, and early cancer in Barrett's oesophagus. Aliment Pharmacol Ther 2006;23:735–42.
53. Hoffman A, Kiesslich R, Bender A, et al. Acetic acid-guided biopsies after magnifying endoscopy compared with random biopsies in the detection of Barrett's esophagus: a prospective randomized trial with crossover design. Gastrointest Endosc 2006;64:1–8.
54. Yagi K, Aruga Y, Nakamura A, et al. The study of dynamic chemical magnifying endoscopy in gastric neoplasia. Gastrointest Endosc 2005;62:963–9.
55. Tanaka K, Toyoda H, Kadowaki S, et al. Features of early gastric cancer and gastric adenoma by enhanced-magnification endoscopy. J Gastroenterol 2006;41:332–8.
56. Yamashita H, Kitayama J, Ishigami H, et al. Endoscopic instillation of indigo carmine dye with acetic acid enables the visualization of distinct margin of superficial gastric lesion; usefulness in endoscopic treatment and diagnosis of gastric cancer. Dig Liver Dis 2007;39:389–92.
57. Togashi K, Hewett DG, Whitaker DA, et al. The use of acetic acid in magnification chromoendoscopy for pit pattern analysis of small polyps. Endoscopy 2006;38:613–6.
58. Kim JH, Lee SY, Kim BK, et al. Importance of the surrounding colonic mucosa in distinguishing between hyperplastic and adenomatous polyps during acetic acid chromoendoscopy. World J Gastroenterol 2008;14:1903–7.
59. Kawamura YJ, Tagashi K, Sasaki J, et al. Acetic acid spray in colonoscopy: an alternative to chromoendoscopy. Gut 2005;54:313.
60. Chisholm EM, Williams SR, Leung JW, et al. Lugol's iodine dye-enhanced endoscopy in patients with cancer of the oesophagus and head and neck. Eur J Surg Oncol 1992;18:550–2.
61. Okomura T, Aruga H, Inohara H, et al. Endoscopic examination of the upper gastrointestinal tract for the presence of second primary cancers in head and neck cancer patients. Acta Otolaryngol Suppl 1993;501:103–6.
62. Yokoyama A, Ohmori T, Makuuchi H, et al. Successful screening for early esophageal cancer in alcoholics using endoscopy and mucosa iodine staining. Cancer 1995;76:928–34.
63. Meyer V, Burtin P, Bour B, et al. Endoscopic detection of early esophageal cancer in high-risk population: does Lugol staining improve videoendoscopy? Gastrointest Endosc 1997;45:480–4.
64. Fagundes RB, de Barros SG, Putten AC, et al. Occult dysplasia is disclosed by Lugol chromoendoscopy in alcoholics at high risk for squamous cell carcinoma of the esophagus. Endoscopy 1999;31:281–5.
65. Hashimoto CL, Iriya K, Baba ER, et al. Lugol's dye spray chromoendoscopy establishes early diagnosis of esophageal cancer in patients with primary head and neck cancer. Am J Gastroenterol 2005;100:275–82.
66. Dawsey SM, Fleischer DE, Wang GQ, et al. Mucosal iodine staining improves endoscopic visualization of squamous dysplasia and squamous cell carcinoma of the esophagus in Linxian, China. Cancer 1998;83:220–31.
67. Muto M, Hironaka S, Nakane M, et al. Association of multiple Lugol-voiding lesions with synchronous and metachronous esophageal squamous cell

carcinoma in patients with head and neck cancer. Gastrointest Endosc 2002;56: 517–21.
68. Katada C, Muto M, Manabe T, et al. Local recurrence of squamous-cell carcinoma of the esophagus after EMR. Gastrointest Endosc 2005;61:219–25.
69. Shimizu Y, Tukagoshi H, Fujita M, et al. Metachronous squamous cell carcinoma of the esophagus arising after endoscopic mucosal resection. Gastrointest Endosc 2001;54:190–4.
70. Hix WR, Wilson WR. Toluidine blue staining of the esophagus. A useful adjunct in the panendoscopic evaluation of patients with squamous cell carcinoma of the head and neck. Arch Otolaryngol Head Neck Surg 1987;113:864–5.
71. Takeo Y, Yoshida T, Shigemitu T, et al. Endoscopic mucosal resection for early esophageal cancer and esophageal dysplasia. Hepatogastroenterology 2001; 48:453–7.
72. Canto MI. Chromoendoscopy and magnifying endoscopy for Barrett's esophagus. Clin Gastroenterol Hepatol 2005;3(7 Suppl 1):S12–5.
73. Ragunath K, Krasner N, Raman VS, et al. A randomized, prospective cross-over trial comparing methylene blue-directed biopsy and conventional random biopsy for detecting intestinal metaplasia and dysplasia in Barrett's esophagus. Endoscopy 2003;35:998–1003.
74. Canto MI, Setrakian S, Willis JE, et al. Methylene blue staining of dysplastic and nondysplastic Barrett's esophagus: an in vivo and ex vivo study. Endoscopy 2001;33:391–400.
75. Sharma P, Topalovski M, Mayo MS, et al. Methylene blue chromoendoscopy for detection of short-segment Barrett's esophagus. Gastrointest Endosc 2001;54:289–93.
76. Kouklakis GS, Kountouras J, Dokas SM, et al. Methylene blue chromoendoscopy for the detection of Barrett's esophagus in a Greek cohort. Endoscopy 2003;35:383–7.
77. Yagi K, Nakamura A, Sekine A. Accuracy of magnifying endoscopy with methylene blue in the diagnosis of specialized intestinal metaplasia and short-segment Barrett's esophagus in Japanese patients without Helicobacter pylori infection. Gastrointest Endosc 2003;58:189–95.
78. Dave U, Shousha S, Westaby D, et al. Methylene blue staining: is it really useful in Barrett's esophagus? Gastrointest Endosc 2001;53:333–5.
79. Wo JM, Ray MB, Mayfield-Stokes S, et al. Comparison of methylene blue-directed biopsies and conventional biopsies in the detection of intestinal metaplasia and dysplasia in Barrett's esophagus: a preliminary study. Gastrointest Endosc 2001;54:294–301.
80. Egger K, Werner M, Meining A, et al. Biopsy surveillance is still necessary in patients with Barrett's oesophagus despite new endoscopic imaging techniques. Gut 2003;54:18–23.
81. Duncan MB, Horwhat JD, Maydonovitch CL, et al. Use of methylene blue for detection of specialized intestinal metaplasia in GERD patients presenting for screening upper endoscopy. Dig Dis Sci 2005;50:389–93.
82. Breyer HP, Silva de Barros SG, Maguilnik I, et al. Does methylene blue detect intestinal metaplasia in Barrett's esophagus. Gastrointest Endosc 2003;57:505–9.
83. Meining A, Rosch T, Kiesslich R, et al. Inter- and intra-observer variability of magnification chromoendoscopy for detecting specialized intestinal metaplasia at the gastroesophageal junction. Endoscopy 2004;36:160–4.
84. Gossner L, Pech O, May A, et al. Comparison of methylene blue-directed biopsies and four-quadrant biopsies in the detection of high-grade intraepithelial neoplasia and early cancer in Barrett's oesophagus. Dig Liver Dis 2006;38:724–9.

85. Gangarosa LM, Halter S, Mertz H. Methylene blue staining and endoscopic ultrasound evaluation of Barrett's esophagus with low-grade dysplasia. Dig Dis Sci 2000;45:225–9.
86. Lim CH, Rotimi O, Dexter SP, et al. Randomized crossover study that used methylene blue or random 4-quadrant biopsy for the diagnosis of dysplasia in Barrett's esophagus. Gastrointest Endosc 2006;64:195–9.
87. Woolf GM, Riddell RH, Irvine EJ, et al. A study to examine agreement between endoscopy and histology for the diagnosis of columnar lined (Barrett's) esophagus. Gastrointest Endosc 1989;35:541–4.
88. Amano Y, Kushiyama Y, Ishihara S, et al. Crystal violet chromoendoscopy with mucosal pit pattern diagnosis is useful for surveillance of short-segment Barrett's esophagus. Am J Gastroenterol 2005;100:21–6.
89. Mayinger B, Oezturk Y, Stolte M, et al. Evaluation of sensitivity and inter- and intra-observer variability in the detection of intestinal metaplasia and dysplasia in Barrett's esophagus with enhanced magnification endoscopy. Scand J Gastroenterol 2006;41:349–56.
90. Conio M. Esophageal chromoendoscopy in Barrett's esophagus: "cons. Gastrointest Endosc 2006;64:9–12.
91. Kudo S, Tamura S, Nakajima T, et al. Diagnosis of colorectal tumorous lesions by magnifying endoscopy. Gastrointest Endosc 1996;44:8–14.
92. Axelrad A, Fleischer DE, Geller AJ, et al. High-resolution chromoendoscopy for the diagnosis of diminutive colon polyps: implications for colon cancer screening. Gastroenterology 1996;110:1253–8.
93. Togashi K, Konishi F, Ishizuka T, et al. Efficacy of magnifying endoscopy in the differential diagnosis of neoplastic and non-neoplastic polyps of the large bowel. Dis Colon Rectum 1999;42:1602–8.
94. Tung SY, Wu CS, Su MY. Magnifying colonoscopy in differentiating neoplastic from nonneoplastic colorectal lesions. Am J Gastroenterol 2001; 96:2628–32.
95. Kato S, Fukii T, Koba I, et al. Assessment of colorectal lesions using magnifying colonoscopy and mucosal dye spraying; can significant lesions be distinguished? Endoscopy 2001;33:306–10.
96. Eisen GM, Kim CY, Fleischer DE, et al. High-resolution chromoendoscopy for classifying colonic polyps: a multicenter study. Gastrointest Endosc 2002;55: 687–94.
97. Konishi K, Kaneko K, Kurahashi T, et al. A comparison of magnifying and nonmagnifying colonoscopy for diagnosis of colorectal polyps: a prospective study. Gastrointest Endosc 2003;57:48–53.
98. Su MY, Ho YP, Chen PC, et al. Magnifying endoscopy with indigo carmine contrast for differential diagnosis of neoplastic and nonneoplastic colonic polyps. Dig Dis Sci 2004;49:1123–7.
99. Hurlstone DP, Cross SS, Adam I, et al. Efficacy of high magnification chromoscopic colonoscopy for the diagnosis of neoplasia in flat and depressed lesions of the colorectum: a prospective analysis. Gut 2004;53:284–90.
100. Fu KI, Sano Y, Kato S, et al. Chromoendoscopy using indigo carmine dye spraying with magnifying observation is the most reliable method for differential diagnosis between non-neoplastic and neoplastic colorectal lesions: a prospective study. Endoscopy 2004;36:1089–93.
101. Apel D, Jakobs R, Schilling D, et al. Accuracy of high-resolution chromoendoscopy in prediction of histologic findings in diminutive lesions of the rectosigmoid. Gastrointest Endosc 2006;63:824–8.

102. Huang Q, Fukami N, Kashida H, et al. Interobserver and intra-observer consistency in the endoscopic assessment of colonic pit patterns. Gastrointest Endosc 2004;60:520–6.
103. Rembacken BJ, Fujii T, Cairns A, et al. Flat and depressed colonic neoplasms: a prospective study of 1000 colonoscopies in the UK. Lancet 2000;355:1211–4.
104. Lee JH, Kim JW, Cho YK, et al. Detection of colorectal adenomas by routine chromoendoscopy with indigocarmine. Am J Gastroenterol 2003;98:1284–8.
105. Soetikno RM, Kaltenbach T, Rouse RV, et al. Prevalence of nonpolypoid (flat and depressed) colorectal neoplasms in asymptomatic and symptomatic adults. JAMA 2008;299:1027–35.
106. Brooker JC, Saunders BP, Shah SG, et al. Total colonic dye-spray increases the detection of diminutive adenomas during routine colonoscopy; a randomized controlled trial. Gastrointest Endosc 2002;56:333–8.
107. Le Rhun M, Coron E, Parlier D, et al. High resolution colonoscopy with chromoscopy versus standard colonoscopy for the detection of colonic neoplasia: a randomized study. Clin Gastroenterol Hepatol 2006;4:349–54.
108. Hurlstone DP, Cross SS, Slater R, et al. Detecting diminutive colorectal lesions at colonoscopy: a randomized controlled trial of pan-colonic versus targeted chromoendoscopy. Gut 2004;53:376–80.
109. Lecomte T, Cellier C, Meatchi T, et al. Chromoendoscopic colonoscopy for detecting preneoplastic lesions in hereditary nonpolyposis colorectal cancer syndrome. Clin Gastroenterol Hepatol 2005;3:897–902.
110. Hurlstone DP, Karajeh M, Cross SS, et al. The role of high-magnification-chromoscopic colonoscopy in hereditary nonpolyposis colorectal cancer screening: a prospective "back-to-back" endoscopic study. Am J Gastroenterol 2005; 100:2167–73.
111. Hurlstone DP, Brown S, Cross SS, et al. High magnification chromoscopic colonoscopy or high frequency 20 MHz mini probe endoscopic ultrasound staging for early colorectal neoplasia: a comparative prospective analysis. Gut 2005;54:1585–9.
112. Hurlstone DP, Cross SS, Brown S, et al. A prospective evaluation of high-magnification chromoscopic colonoscopy in predicting completeness of EMR. Gastrointest Endosc 2004;59:642–50.
113. Soetikno RM, Gotoda T, Naknishi Y, et al. Endoscopic mucosal resection. Gastrointest Endosc 2003;57:567–79.
114. Kiesslich R, Fritsch J, Holtmann M, et al. Methylene blue-aided chromoendoscopy for the detection of intraepithelial neoplasia and colon cancer in ulcerative colitis. Gastroenterology 2003;124:880–8.
115. Hulrlstone DP, McAlindon ME, Sanders DS, et al. Further validation of high-magnification chromoscopic-colonoscopy for the detection of intraepithelial neoplasia and colon cancer in ulcerative colitis. Gastroenterology 2004;126:376–7.
116. Matsumoto T, Nakamura S, Jo Y, et al. Chromoscopy might improve diagnostic accuracy in cancer surveillance for ulcerative colitis. Am J Gastroenterol 2003;98:1827–33.
117. Rutter MD, Saunders BP, Schofield G, et al. Pancolonic indigo carmine dye spraying for the detection of dysplasia in ulcerative colitis. Gut 2004;53:256–60.
118. Hurlstone DP, Sanders DS, Lobo AJ, et al. Indigo carmine-assisted high-magnification chromoscopic colonoscopy for the detection and characterisation of intraepithelial neoplasia in ulcerative colitis: a prospective evaluation. Endoscopy 2005;37:1186–92.
119. Sada M, Igarashi M, Yoshizawa S, et al. Dye spraying and magnifying endoscopy for dysplasia and cancer surveillance in ulcerative colitis. Dis Colon Rectum 2004;47:1816–23.

Autofluorescence Endoscopy

Gary W. Falk, MD, MS

KEYWORDS

- Autofluorescence endoscopy • Barrett's esophagus
- Dysplasia • Esophageal adenocarcinoma
- Endoscopic surveillance

Autofluorescence endoscopy is a wide-area imaging technique, with the ability to rapidly examine a large surface area of gastrointestinal mucosa to detect small areas of dysplasia or cancer. It has potential in diseases such as Barrett's esophagus, ulcerative colitis and gastric cancer, in which large areas of mucosa may harbor areas of dysplasia or superficial cancer not visible on conventional or high-definition white-light endoscopy. This article examines the rationale for this technology and the data to date on fiberoptic and video autofluorescence endoscopy. Most of the work in this field has been on Barrett's esophagus surveillance, which is used as the conceptual model for autofluorescence endoscopy throughout this article.

THE CLINICAL PROBLEM

Endoscopic surveillance is used for premalignant diseases such as Barrett's esophagus, ulcerative colitis, and, in high-risk areas of the world, chronic gastritis. For each of these diseases, dysplasia and early carcinoma may be invisible with standard or high-definition white-light imaging. Current endoscopic surveillance programs rely on high-resolution or high-definition white-light endoscopy. For Barrett's esophagus, practice guidelines suggest obtaining systematic four quadrant biopsies at 2-cm intervals along the entire length of the Barrett's segment.[1] The rationale for such a comprehensive biopsy program comes from observations that high-grade dysplasia and early carcinoma in Barrett's esophagus often occur in the absence of endoscopic abnormalities, and from the focal nature of dysplasia. Systematic esophagectomy mapping studies demonstrate just how focal dysplasia and superficial cancer may be.[2] In 30 esophagectomy specimens from patients undergoing surgery for either high-grade dysplasia or early invasive adenocarcinoma with no endoscopic evidence of cancer, the median surface area of total Barrett's esophagus was found to be 32 cm^2; low-grade dysplasia 13 cm^2; high-grade dysplasia 1.3 cm^2; and adenocarcinoma 1.1 cm^2. The 3 smallest cancers had surface areas of 0.02, 0.3 and 0.4 cm^2.

Department of Gastroenterology and Hepatology, Cleveland Clinic Lerner College of Medicine of Case Western Reserve University, Desk A-31, Cleveland Clinic, 9500 Euclid Avenue, Cleveland, OH 44195, USA
E-mail address: falkg@ccf.org

Gastrointest Endoscopy Clin N Am 19 (2009) 209–220
doi:10.1016/j.giec.2009.02.004 giendo.theclinics.com
1052-5157/09/$ – see front matter

Endoscopic surveillance of Barrett's esophagus, as currently practiced, has numerous shortcomings. Dysplasia and early adenocarcinoma are endoscopically indistinguishable from intestinal metaplasia without dysplasia. The distribution of dysplasia and cancer is highly variable, and even the most thorough biopsy surveillance program has the potential for sampling error. There are considerable interobserver variability and quality control problems in the interpretation of dysplasia in community and academic settings.[3]

To make surveillance techniques more effective, new approaches are necessary. More effective surveillance techniques can be accomplished conceptually by optically sampling larger areas of Barrett's mucosa and targeting biopsies to areas with a higher probability of harboring dysplasia. A variety of endoscopic techniques have attempted to improve the efficiency and sampling in surveillance programs. The goals of optical enhancements to current white-light endoscopy include (1) increased efficiency of tissue sampling for detection of high risk lesions, (2) the ability to target biopsies at highest risk mucosa, (3) decrease the number of biopsies, and (4) decrease the overall costs of endoscopic surveillance.[4] All of these techniques are based on the principle that benign and malignant tissues have different optical qualities.

PRINCIPLES OF AUTOFLUORESCENCE ENDOSCOPY

Autofluorescence endoscopy is a technique that allows wide-area imaging of the mucosa of the gastrointestinal tract. The goal of this red-flag technology is to define areas of dysplasia or neoplasia not visible with white-light endoscopy, thereby allowing for targeted biopsies of high-risk mucosa. In theory, this technique has the potential to rapidly assess large areas of epithelium before targeting biopsies without the need to administer exogenous substances to the patient to detect tissue fluorescence. To date, the technique has been applied to the esophagus, stomach, and colon, with much of the work taking place in the esophagus.

Autofluorescence endoscopy involves illumination of the tissue of interest with short wavelength (ie, blue) light, which leads to excitation of endogenous substances known as fluorophores and hence emission of fluorescent light of longer wavelength.[5] It is based on the principal that tissue excited by light of a specific wavelength will emit fluorescent light of a longer wavelength, and that normal, metaplastic, and dysplastic tissues have different autofluorescence colors visible to the naked eye.[5] Fluorophores responsible for tissue autofluorescence include collagen, porphyrins, aromatic amino acids, flavins, and reduced nicotinamide adenine dinucleotide (NADH), with collagen being the most important contributor to tissue autofluorescence in the gastrointestinal tract. Other molecules known as chromophores can absorb excitation light and fluorescence light; hemoglobin is the best example of such a substance. Because the sources of fluorescence are endogenous to the tissue of interest, the fluorescence is termed autofluorescence.

Autofluorescence endoscopy takes advantage of the difference in concentration of endogenous fluorophores to help differentiate dysplastic and neoplastic epithelium from normal mucosa. It has the advantage of avoiding the use of exogenous contrast agents. The reason that normal, metaplastic, and dysplastic epithelial structures have different autofluorescence characteristics is related to the type, concentration, and distribution of the various chromophores and fluorophores along with the morphologic changes in cell structure that occur during disease progression. This interplay between exciting light, biochemical composition of the target tissue, and tissue perfusion determines the autofluorescence appearance of the mucosal surface.[6] In Barrett's epithelium, it is believed that 3 underlying mechanisms account for the difference in autofluorescence between benign and neoplastic epithelium:[7] (1) neoplastic cells have an increased nuclear to cytoplasmic ratio, with a reduction in autofluorescence due to the fact that little autofluorescence comes from the nuclei; (2) the mucosal layer thickens, often due to increased collagen deposition and hence decreased autofluorescence; (3) alterations in blood flow during neoplastic transformation lead to increased absorption of fluorescence. As such, neoplasia should result in less autofluorescence than nonneoplastic tissue.

FIBEROPTIC SYSTEMS

Early work with autofluorescence endoscopy involved fiberoptic technology with a specially designed overhead camera that allowed switching back and forth between the white-light image and the autofluorescence image. These systems involved transmission of fluorescence by fiberoptic bundles to the proximal end of an endoscope for spectral filtering. Two systems have been developed. One is the light-induced fluorescence endoscopy (LIFE) system (Xillix Technologies Corp, Richmond, BC, Canada), which consists of a fiberoptic endoscope with a camera attached that allows rapid switching between white-light and autofluorescence modes. The LIFE system uses blue light at a wavelength of 400 to 450 nm to stimulate autofluorescence.[8] Two charged couple device (CCD) cameras attached to the fiberoptic endoscope by way of a detachable module are used to capture red and green autofluorescence signals (**Fig. 1**). These signals are then fused to create a composite pseudocolor image in which normal tissue appears green and abnormal tissue appears red. This system permits rapid switching between conventional white-light images and autofluorescence images. Unfortunately, this system is bulky, making manipulation challenging. The other fiberoptic system, D-Light (Storz Ltd., Tuttlingen, Germany), has been used primarily for fluorescence induced by 5-aminolevulinic acid.

Haringsma and colleagues[9] demonstrated the potential of the LIFE II system in a proof-of-principle case series of four patients. Two patients with Barrett's esophagus had areas of high-grade dysplasia, which were seen as areas of red fluorescence in areas of subtle white-light imaging changes. One patient had signet cell cancer of the stomach demonstrated by dark red areas in the stomach; a second patient had a flat area clearly seen by autofluorescence endoscopy but not well seen by white-light endoscopy, which was found to be an adenoma.

Niepsuj and colleagues[10] examined the efficacy of the LIFE system in a study of 34 patients with short segment Barrett's esophagus. This system results in reddish-brown fluorescence in the Barrett's epithelium compared with background green fluorescence in the squamous epithelium. In some of the patients there were qualitatively more intense areas of red fluorescence within the Barrett's epithelium, which were targeted for biopsy. High-grade dysplasia was found in nine (8.3%) autofluorescence-guided biopsy specimens compared with one of the white-light–guided biopsy specimens (0.7%). Thus, autofluorescence endoscopy resulted in the detection of high-grade dysplasia in 7 of 34 patients (21%) versus 1 of 34 patients (3%) with white-light endoscopy. There was no difference between autofluorescence-guided biopsies and random white-light–guided biopsies for the detection of low-grade dysplasia. These findings offer promise for the role of autofluorescence endoscopy as a wide-field, red-flag technology for the detection of dysplasia in Barrett's esophagus.

Another case series of Barrett's esophagus patients reported by Egger and colleagues,[11] using the LIFE system, found the sensitivity of this technique for the diagnosis of cancer or dysplasia to be only 37% with a specificity of 91%. In 35 patients, autofluorescence endoscopy detected one additional case of high-grade

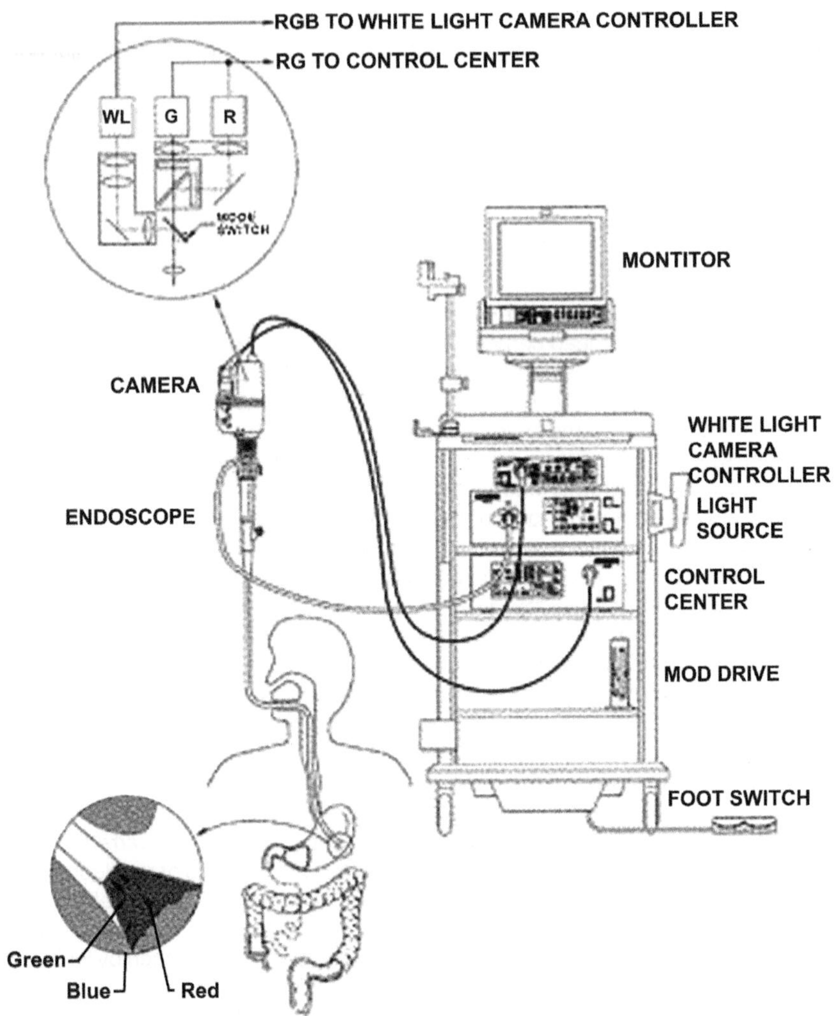

Fig. 1. The LIFE II system. (*From* Haringsma J, Tytgat GN, Yano H, et al. Autofluorescence endoscopy: feasibility of detection of GI neoplasms unapparent to white light endoscopy with an evolving technology. Gastrointest Endosc 2001;53:642–50; with permission.)

dysplasia and seven additional areas of low-grade dysplasia (**Fig. 2**). Borovicka and colleagues[12] found that of 19 lesions with high-grade dysplasia or adenocarcinoma, autofluorescence endoscopy with the Storz system detected only eight for a sensitivity of 42%, whereas random biopsies picked up the other 11 lesions. Kara and colleagues[13] performed a randomized crossover trial of the LIFE-II autofluorescence endoscopy versus white-light video endoscopy in 47 patients with Barrett's esophagus and could find no difference in the detection rates for high-grade dysplasia or adenocarcinoma between the two techniques (**Fig. 3**). Acute inflammation was present more often in false positive lesions than in true negative lesions by autofluorescence endoscopy.

The LIFE system has also been evaluated in gastric neoplasia. Ohkawa and colleagues[14] found that the sensitivity of autofluorescence endoscopy for neoplastic

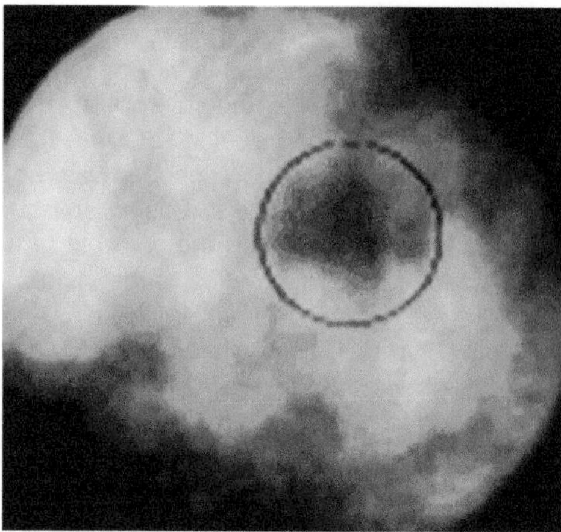

Fig. 2. Patient with Barrett's esophagus and biopsy-proven high-grade dysplasia visible only on fiberoptic autofluorescence endoscopy but not on white-light video endoscopy. (*From* Egger K, Werner M, Meining A, et al. Biopsy surveillance is still necessary in patients with Barrett's oesophagus despite new endoscopic imaging techniques. Gut 2003;52:18–23; with permission.)

lesions was 96.4% (54/56), whereas 49.1% (26/53) of benign lesions had an abnormal autofluorescence pattern.

Overall, this technique has limited clinical value because of poor image quality related to the use of fiberoptic technology for the white-light and autofluorescence endoscopy images in the current era of video endoscopy, along with the problem of poor maneuverability of the bulky imaging platform.

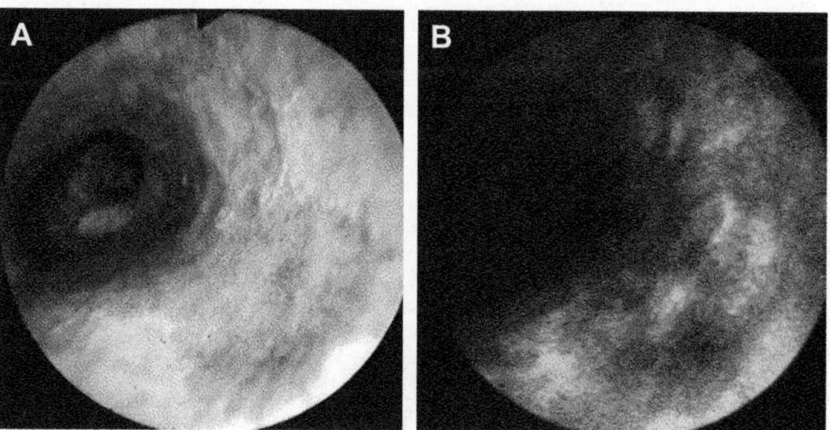

Fig. 3. (*A*) White-light fiberoptic endoscopic image of the proximal end of a segment of Barrett's esophagus. (*B*) Corresponding light-induced autofluorescence endoscopic image showing a false positive area proximally. Biopsy specimens from this area were found to contain intestinal metaplasia without dysplasia on review. (*From* Kara MA, Smits ME, Rosmolen WD, et al. A randomized crossover study comparing light-induced fluorescence endoscopy with standard video endoscopy for the detection of early neoplasia in Barrett's esophagus. Gastrointest Endosc 2005;61:671–8; with permission.)

VIDEO SYSTEMS

More recently, this technique has been adapted to video technology with a considerable improvement in image quality. Unlike the fiberoptic system, the initial video technology incorporated a charge-coupled device (CCD) in the distal tip instead of the handle of the endoscope and autofluorescence was combined with green (540–560 nm) and red (600–620 nm) reflectance.[15] This improved the quality and resolution of the autofluorescence image, improved the contrast of the image, and most importantly, improved the handling characteristics of the instrument, compared with the fiberoptic techniques.

The initial Olympus system (Olympus, Tokyo, Japan) has the following components: a red, green, blue sequential light source, a high-resolution video endoscope and two CCD chips, one of which is used for white-light imaging and the other for autofluorescence imaging (**Fig. 4**).[16] Fluorescence images are composed sequentially from pseudocolors from three components: total autofluorescence in response to blue light excitation (395–475 nm); red reflectance light (600–620 nm); and green reflectance light (540–560 nm). Light is provided by a xenon lamp and fluorescence detection (490–625 nm) is detected at the CCD.[17] With this system, dysplasia and cancer in Barrett's esophagus appears purple/magenta compared with the green appearance of nondysplastic mucosa.

The differences between the video and fiberoptic systems are summarized in **Table 1**.[15] Resolution with the video system is due to the number of pixels in the CCD detector, which is approximately tenfold greater than the fiberoptic system. The signal-to-noise ratio is enhanced with the video system because fluorescence is detected immediately past the objective lens, whereas the fiberoptic detection requires transmission through bundles to an image intensifier. Video contrast is superior to fiberoptic contrast and the video system can detect the white-light image and autofluorescence using the same CCD in contrast to the fiberoptic system, which

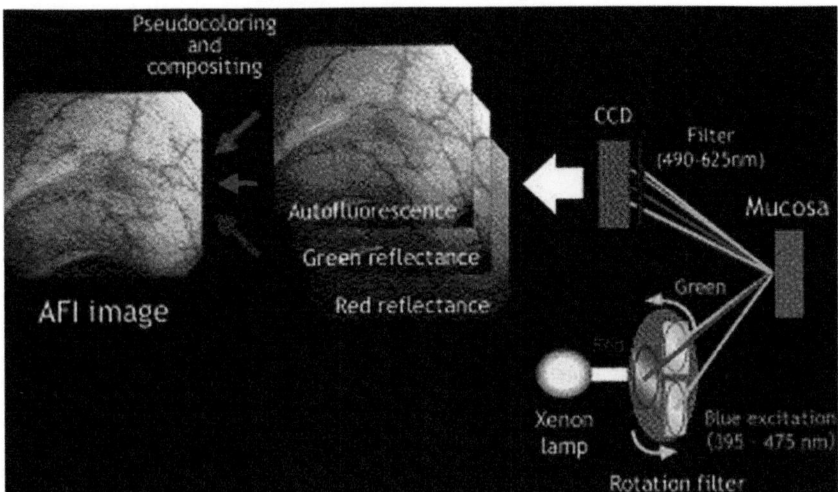

Fig. 4. Principles of the video autofluorescence endoscopy system. Autofluorescence, and green and red reflectance images are pseudocolored to form a composite autofluorescence endoscopy image. AFI, autofluorescence imaging. (*From* Uedo N, Iishi H, Tatsuta M, et al. A novel videoendoscopy system by using autofluorescence and reflectance imaging for diagnosis of esophagogastric cancers. Gastrointest Endosc 2005;62:521–8; with permission.)

Table 1
Imaging parameters comparing fiberoptic and video autofluorescence imaging systems

Image Parameter	Video	Fiberoptic
Resolution elements	~100,000	~10,000
Intensifier	No	Yes
Contrast	Higher	Lower
Registration	Complete	Incomplete
Spectral filtering	Fixed	Flexible

Data from Wang TD, Triadafilopoulos G. Autofluorescence imaging: have we finally seen the light? Gastrointest Endosc 2005;61:686–8.

requires separate CCDs. On the other hand, the fiberoptic system has flexible spectral filtering in contrast to the fixed filtering in the video system.

Initial work by Uedo and colleagues[18] with the Olympus video system found that autofluorescence endoscopy correctly detected the extent of superficial esophageal carcinoma in five out of five patients, whereas white-light imaging correctly identified the lesion extent in only two of the five patients. For superficial gastric carcinoma, autofluorescence endoscopy correctly determined lesion extent in 15 of 22 (68%) of cases compared with 8 of 22 (36%) with white-light endoscopy.

Kara and colleagues[19] examined 60 patients with Barrett's esophagus using high-resolution white-light video endoscopy and autofluorescence endoscopy. High-grade dysplasia or early carcinoma was detected in 22 patients of whom only one had no visible white-light abnormality. Of the 21 patients with a visible lesion, high-grade dysplasia or carcinoma was detectable by either white-light endoscopy or autofluorescence endoscopy. However, in six patients, the lesions were detectable only with autofluorescence endoscopy and not with white-light endoscopy (**Fig. 5**). The detection rate of high-grade dysplasia or cancer increased from 23% to 33% of patients using autofluorescence endoscopy and the total number of lesions detected

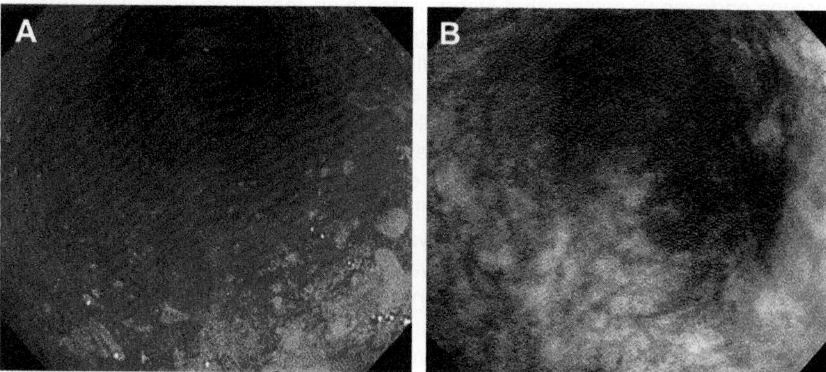

Fig. 5. A true positive autofluorescence endoscopy image using a video endoscopy system. (*A*) White-light image reveals no evidence of mucosal abnormality. (*B*) Autofluorescence endoscopy image reveals blue purple color on the right-hand side. Biopsies from the abnormal area revealed adenocarcinoma. (*From* Kara MA, Peters FP, Ten Kate FJ, et al. Endoscopic video autofluorescence imaging may improve the detection of early neoplasia in patients with Barrett's esophagus. Gastrointest Endosc 2005;61:679–85; with permission.)

increased from 20 to 40. However, autofluorescence endoscopy was still associated with a high number of false positive areas of abnormal fluorescence. In this study, 28 of 81 regions (35%) of abnormal fluorescence were associated with no dysplasia. Thus, the positive predictive value was 49% and the negative predictive value was 89%. In contrast to the true negative samples, the false positive areas were characterized by more prominent acute inflammatory changes. In a screening test such as this, it is essential that false negative findings are minimized.

One case report has been published using the Olympus video autofluorescence endoscopy system in cancer surveillance of ulcerative colitis.[20]

TRIMODAL SYSTEMS

In an effort to decrease the high false positive rates found with autofluorescence endoscopy when used as a stand-alone technique, Kara and colleagues combined autofluorescence endoscopy with narrow band imaging in a series of studies. They performed a proof-of-principle study in which autofluorescence video endoscopy was used as a red-flag technique to identify suspicious areas of Barrett's mucosa, followed by narrow band imaging combined with magnification endoscopy to examine the vascular and mucosal pattern of these suspicious lesions.[21] This study was performed with two prototype endoscopes (Olympus Inc., Tokyo, Japan): one with autofluorescence endoscopy and high-resolution white-light video endoscopy as described earlier and the other with narrow band imaging with magnification and white-light video endoscopy. Twenty patients referred for management of high-grade dysplasia had a total of 28 biopsy-proven lesions. Autofluorescence endoscopy detected all of these lesions; 11 (40%) were detected only by autofluorescence endoscopy. However, there were 19 other abnormalities detected by autofluorescence endoscopy that did not have high-grade dysplasia, giving a false positive rate of 40%. Narrow band imaging revealed no suspicious changes in 14 of these 19 lesions, which reduced the false positive rate to 10% of the original 47 lesions. These results suggested that the combination of these two techniques had the potential to improve the performance characteristics of autofluorescence endoscopy.

This led to work by Curvers and colleagues,[22] from the same group, with a novel prototype endoscope system that incorporated high-resolution white-light autofluorescence endoscopy and narrow band imaging with optical zoom into one endoscope. In this system (Olympus Inc.), the autofluorescence image is composed of total emitted autofluorescence after blue light excitation (390–470 nm) and green reflectance (540–560 nm) unlike the previous video system in which the image consisted of total autofluorescence, red reflectance, and green reflectance. This multicenter study examined a more diverse group of 84 patients with Barrett's esophagus including those undergoing routine surveillance and those being managed for endoscopically indistinguishable high-grade dysplasia or superficial cancer. A total of 30 patients were found to have biopsy-proven intramucosal carcinoma or high-grade dysplasia. Autofluorescence endoscopy increased the detection rate from 16 of 30 (45%) by white light alone to 27 of 30 (90%). Autofluorescence endoscopy also increased the total number of biopsy-proven lesions with intramucosal carcinoma or high-grade dysplasia from 21 with high-resolution white light alone to 40 with autofluorescence endoscopy after white light. Autofluorescence endoscopy detected 102 lesions not seen with high-resolution white-light endoscopy, of which 83 (81%) did not have high-grade dysplasia or intramucosal carcinoma. Narrow band imaging reduced the false positive rate from 81% to 26%, again supporting the concept of trimodal imaging (**Figs. 6** and **7**). These two studies demonstrate the promise of

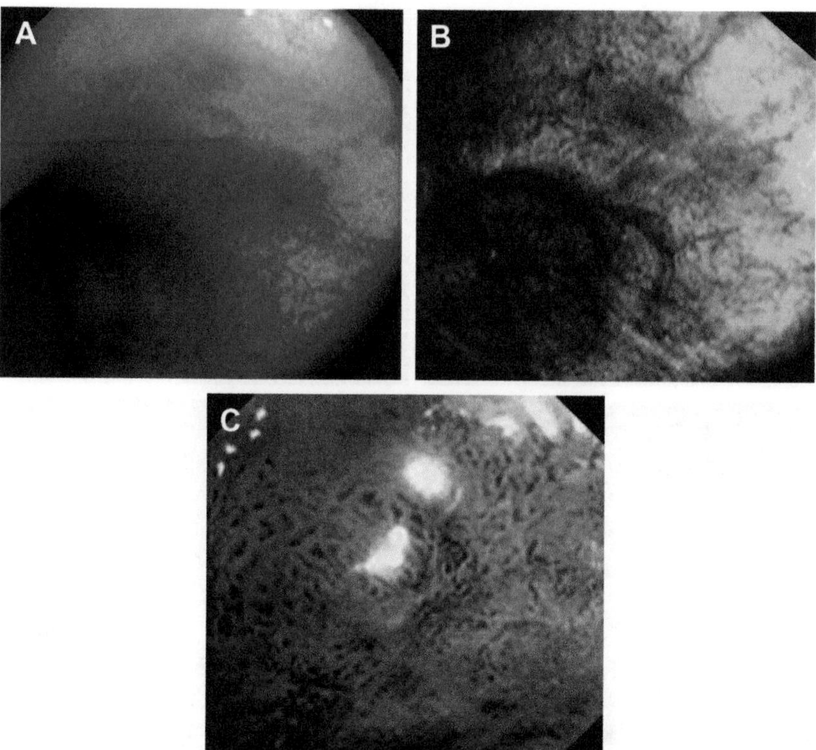

Fig. 6. True positive autofluorescence endoscopy with trimodal imaging system. (*A*) Normal white-light endoscopy image; (*B*) suspicious area of purple autofluorescence at the 1 o'clock position; (*C*) narrow band image shows irregular mucosal and vascular patterns. Histology demonstrated adenocarcinoma. (*From* Curvers WL, Singh R, Song LM, et al. Endoscopic tri-modal imaging for detection of early neoplasia in Barrett's oesophagus: a multi-centre feasibility study using high-resolution endoscopy, autofluorescence imaging and narrow band imaging incorporated in one endoscopy system. Gut 2008;57:167–72; with permission.)

autofluorescence endoscopy when combined with narrow band imaging and high-resolution white-light endoscopy for surveillance of Barrett's esophagus. However, both of these studies were performed in tertiary care centers by experienced endoscopists on patients at high risk for high-grade dysplasia and early carcinoma.

LIMITATIONS OF CURRENT TECHNOLOGY

Unfortunately, despite the conceptual simplicity of autofluorescence endoscopy to provide enhanced endoscopic imaging, the technology in its current version is limited. First, image quality with the current video systems, although better than earlier fiberoptic systems, is still inferior to high-resolution and high-definition white-light endoscopy. Improved resolution video endoscopy is clearly desirable. Second, the technique only examines surface mucosa and does not allow for visualization of subsurface changes. Deeper tissue penetration would be desirable. Third, the false positive rate remains far too high for autofluorescence endoscopy to be used as a stand-alone technique. The false positive rate may have two components: one is a limitation of the technology alone and another is related to image interpretation

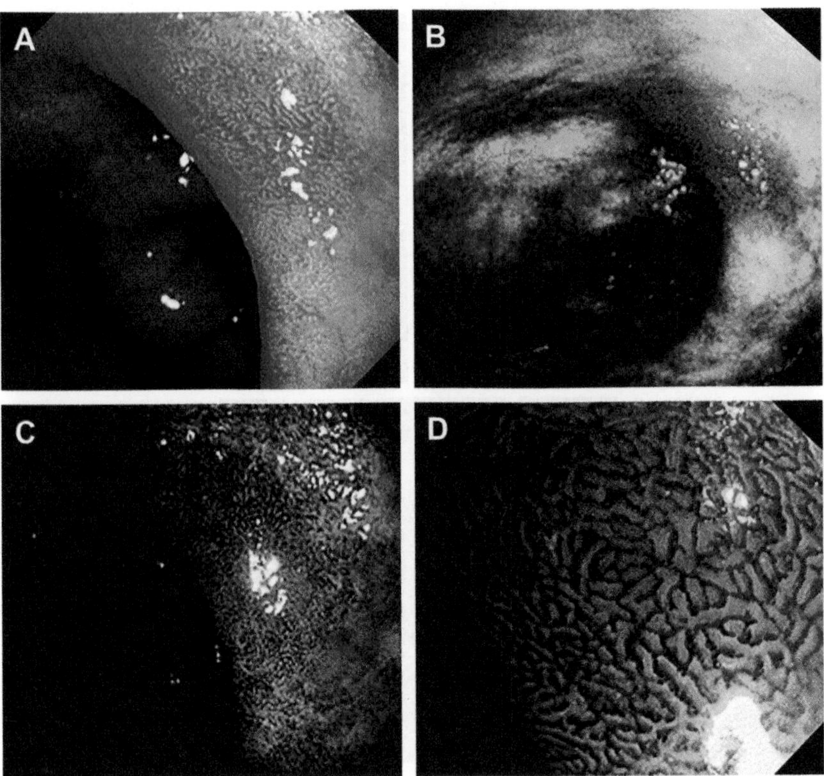

Fig. 7. False positive autofluorescence endoscopy with trimodal imaging system. (*A*) Normal white-light endoscopy image; (*B*) suspicious area of purple autofluorescence at the 2 o'clock position; (*C, D*) narrow band image shows regular mucosal and vascular patterns. Histology demonstrated intestinal metaplasia without dysplasia. (*From* Curvers WL, Singh R, Song LM, et al. Endoscopic tri-modal imaging for detection of early neoplasia in Barrett's oesophagus: a multi-centre feasibility study using high-resolution endoscopy, autofluorescence imaging and narrow band imaging incorporated in one endoscopy system. Gut 2008;57:167–72; with permission.)

relative to movement of the organ of interest as well as distance between the endoscope and the area of interest. As described earlier, combining autofluorescence imaging with a second modality such as narrow band imaging improves the performance characteristics. Fourth, the color tone is unstable and influenced by various conditions including distance from the surface, instrument angulation, and air insufflation. Finally, autofluorescence technology detects indirect measures of dysplasia and carcinoma and is therefore nonspecific.

SUMMARY

Autofluorescence endoscopy offers a conceptual paradigm for wide-area imaging to allow for targeted biopsies so desirable in endoscopic surveillance programs. Fiberoptic systems are no longer tenable due to poor image quality in a world accustomed to high-definition quality images. Although current video technology has improved the quality of images, there are still too many false positives to make this tool useful as a stand-alone technique in clinical practice. Additional improvements are still needed in fluorescence image quality. Studies using trimodal imaging offer great promise but require additional validation.

REFERENCES

1. Wang KK, Sampliner RE. Practice Parameters Committee of the American College of Gastroenterology. Updated guidelines 2008 for the diagnosis, surveillance and therapy of Barrett's esophagus. Am J Gastroenterol 2008;103:788–97.
2. Cameron AJ, Carpenter HA. Barrett's esophagus, high-grade dysplasia, and early adenocarcinoma: a pathological study. Am J Gastroenterol 1997;92(4): 586–91.
3. Montgomery E, Bronner MP, Goldblum JR, et al. Reproducibility of the diagnosis of dysplasia in Barrett esophagus: a reaffirmation. Hum Pathol 2001;32:368–78.
4. Wang TD, Van Dam J. Optical biopsy: a new frontier in endoscopic detection and diagnosis. Clin Gastroenterol Hepatol 2004;2:744–53.
5. Kara MA, DaCosta RS, Streutker CJ, et al. Characterization of tissue autofluorescence in Barrett's esophagus by confocal fluorescence microscopy. Dis Esophagus 2007;20:141–50.
6. Kara MA, Bergman JJ. Autofluorescence imaging and narrow-band imaging for the detection of early neoplasia in patients with Barrett's esophagus. Endoscopy 2006;38:627–31.
7. Kara M, DaCosta RS, Wilson BC, et al. Autofluorescence-based detection of early neoplasia in patients with Barrett's esophagus. Dig Dis 2004;22:134–41.
8. Ell C. Improving endoscopic resolution and sampling: fluorescence techniques. Gut 2003;52(Suppl 4):iv30–3.
9. Haringsma J, Tytgat GN, Yano H, et al. Autofluorescence endoscopy: feasibility of detection of GI neoplasms unapparent to white light endoscopy with an evolving technology. Gastrointest Endosc 2001;53:642–50.
10. Niepsuj K, Niepsuj G, Cebula W, et al. Autofluorescence endoscopy for detection of high-grade dysplasia in short-segment Barrett's esophagus. Gastrointest Endosc 2003;58:715–9.
11. Egger K, Werner M, Meining A, et al. Biopsy surveillance is still necessary in patients with Barrett's oesophagus despite new endoscopic imaging techniques. Gut 2003;52:18–23.
12. Borovicka J, Fischer J, Neuweiler J, et al. Autofluorescence endoscopy in surveillance of Barrett's esophagus: a multicenter randomized trial on diagnostic efficacy. Endoscopy 2006;38:867–72.
13. Kara MA, Smits ME, Rosmolen WD, et al. A randomized crossover study comparing light-induced fluorescence endoscopy with standard videoendoscopy for the detection of early neoplasia in Barrett's esophagus. Gastrointest Endosc 2005;61:671–8.
14. Ohkawa A, Miwa H, Namihisa A, et al. Diagnostic performance of light-induced fluorescence endoscopy for gastric neoplasms. Endoscopy 2004;36:515–21.
15. Wang TD, Triadafilopoulos G. Autofluorescence imaging: have we finally seen the light? Gastrointest Endosc 2005;61:686–8.
16. Wong Kee Song LM, Wilson BC. Optical detection of high-grade dysplasia in Barrett's esophagus. Tech Gastrointest Endosc 2005;7:78–88.
17. Wong Kee Song LM, Wilson BC. Endoscopic detection of early upper GI cancers. Best Pract Res Clin Gastroenterol 2005;19:833–56.

18. Uedo N, Iishi H, Tatsuta M, et al. A novel videoendoscopy system by using autofluorescence and reflectance imaging for diagnosis of esophagogastric cancers. Gastrointest Endosc 2005;62:521–8.
19. Kara MA, Peters FP, Ten Kate FJ, et al. Endoscopic video autofluorescence imaging may improve the detection of early neoplasia in patients with Barrett's esophagus. Gastrointest Endosc 2005;61:679–85.
20. Matsumoto T, Moriyama T, Yao T, et al. Autofluorescence imaging colonoscopy for the diagnosis of dysplasia in ulcerative colitis. Inflamm Bowel Dis 2007;13:640–1.
21. Kara MA, Peters FP, Fockens P, et al. Endoscopic video-autofluorescence imaging followed by narrow band imaging for detecting early neoplasia in Barrett's esophagus. Gastrointest Endosc 2006;64:176–85.
22. Curvers WL, Singh R, Song LM, et al. Endoscopic tri-modal imaging for detection of early neoplasia in Barrett's oesophagus: a multi-centre feasibility study using high-resolution endoscopy, autofluorescence imaging and narrow band imaging incorporated in one endoscopy system. Gut 2008;57:167–72.

Fluorescence and Raman Spectroscopy

Constantinos P. Anastassiades, MD[a],
Brian C. Wilson, PhD[b], Louis-Michel Wong Kee Song, MD[c,*]

KEYWORDS

• Fluorescence • Raman • Spectroscopy
• Endoscopy • Dysplasia

Optical spectroscopic techniques have the potential to enhance lesion diagnosis in real time during endoscopy. These techniques are based on the analysis of specific light-tissue interactions, such as fluorescence, elastic scattering, and inelastic (Raman) scattering. These optical signals contain information about the microstructural and/or biochemical content of tissue. Spectral differences in the optical signals have been shown to correlate with particular histopathological diagnoses, and they have been exploited for lesion diagnosis or differentiation in the gastrointestinal (GI) tract. Several promising applications include the optical detection of dysplastic and early cancerous lesions in Barrett's esophagus and stomach and the differentiation of colorectal polyps.[1,2]

Similar to standard pinch biopsy, point spectroscopic diagnosis is limited by the small sampling volume (~1 mm^3) and random sampling approach. However, the sampling yield is increased since multiple "optical biopsies" can be collected in the same time interval necessary to obtain a single pinch biopsy. Although point spectroscopic devices obviously cannot compete with their imaging counterparts (eg, autofluorescence imaging) for wide-field mucosal surface assessment, they are nevertheless likely to provide more detailed and specific information about the tissue state and still be useful either as standalone or as adjunctive techniques to other imaging modalities (multimodal approach).

In this article, the current status and future prospects of fluorescence and Raman point spectroscopic devices are discussed as they pertain to endoscopic applications. The related optical imaging techniques (eg, autofluorescence endoscopy) are addressed separately in accompanying reviews.

[a] Division of Gastroenterology, University of Michigan, 3912 Taubman Center, SPC 5362, 1500 E. Medical Center Drive, Ann Arbor, MI 48109, USA
[b] Department of Medical Biophysics, Ontario Cancer Institute/Princess Margaret Hospital, 610 University Avenue, Toronto, Ontario M5G 2M9, Canada
[c] Division of Gastroenterology and Hepatology, Mayo Clinic, 200 First Street S.W., Rochester, MN 55905, USA
* Corresponding author.
E-mail address: wong.louis@mayo.edu (L-M. Wong Kee Song).

Gastrointest Endoscopy Clin N Am 19 (2009) 221–231
doi:10.1016/j.giec.2009.02.009 giendo.theclinics.com
1052-5157/09/$ – see front matter

SPECTROSCOPIC EQUIPMENT

The basic components of a probe-based spectroscopic device are shown in **Fig. 1**. The light source that is selected for tissue excitation depends, in part, on the detection of optical signals of interest. For example, a laser- or wavelength-filtered lamp in the violet-blue spectral range is typically used for excitation of tissue fluorescence, whereas near-infrared laser light excitation is suitable for tissue Raman measurements at endoscopy.

The light source is coupled to a fiber-optic probe, which is inserted into the accessory channel of the endoscope and positioned in close proximity to or in contact with the tissue surface. The probe consists of one or more optical fibers to deliver the excitation light to tissue and collect the emitted optical signals from tissue. The collected signals are relayed to a spectrograph, which disperses the light into its component wavelengths and associated intensities, and are displayed as optical spectra (**Fig. 2**) on a computer monitor.

A fluorescence optical biopsy forceps (*Wav*STAT system, SpectraScience Inc., Minneapolis, Minnesota) has been described in which an optical fiber is incorporated into a standard biopsy forceps, enabling precise pinch biopsy of the probed site immediately following optical measurements.

SPECTRAL ANALYSIS

The methods used for analyzing optical spectra have ranged from simple mathematical algorithms, such as intensity ratios at selected wavelength regions, to advanced multivariate statistical or computational techniques, such as principal component analysis and artificial neural networks. Regardless of the technique employed, the objective is to sort out spectral differences that discriminate between tissue types and to develop classification algorithms based on these spectral differences.

In the absence of objective, well-validated, and widely used molecular biomarkers of cancer risk for premalignant GI conditions, such as Barrett's esophagus, spectral classification algorithms have been developed using histologic diagnosis as the gold standard, albeit an imperfect one. Moreover, as a result of sample size limitations in most spectroscopic studies published to date, statistical resampling techniques, such as leave-one-out or bootstrap-based cross-validation, have been used to *estimate* the sensitivity, specificity, and accuracy of spectral diagnosis relative to histology. Prospective validation regarding the diagnostic performance of fluorescence and Raman classification algorithms using large independent data sets in the GI tract is lacking.

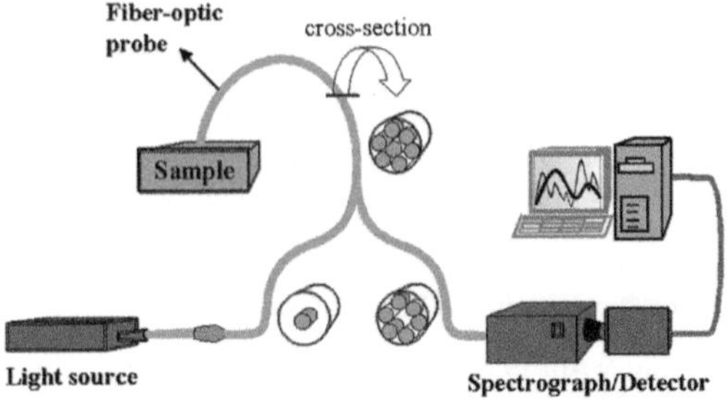

Fig. 1. Simplified setup and basic components of a point spectroscopic system.

FLUORESCENCE SPECTROSCOPY

Principles

Fluorescence refers to the emission of light of longer wavelengths following tissue excitation with a short-wavelength light source. Both naturally occurring tissue fluorescence (autofluorescence) and tissue fluorescence enhanced by the administration of an exogenous agent have been exploited for diagnostic purposes.

Autofluorescence reflects the contributions of several fluorescent biologic molecules (fluorophores) indigenous to tissue (**Table 1**). Following tissue excitation, these fluorophores emit overlapping fluorescence peaks and bands of variable intensities, resulting in a broad and relatively featureless spectral line shape (see **Fig. 2**). Autofluorescence diagnosis is based on detecting differences in spectral line shapes that characterize various tissue types. These spectral differences are a consequence of alterations in fluorophore concentration and/or spatial (eg, depth) distribution, which are associated with biochemical and/or microstructural changes occurring in pathologic tissue.

In the GI tract, autofluorescence spectra typically display a decrease in fluorescence intensity in the green spectral range and a relative increase in red fluorescence, as preneoplastic mucosa, such as Barrett's esophagus, evolves toward carcinoma (**Fig. 3**). In Barrett's esophagus, for example, these spectral differences correlate with observations at the molecular level where low collagen (green) fluorescence associates with lesions containing high-grade dysplasia as opposed to nondysplastic Barrett's epithelia.[3]

The administration of an exogenous fluorophore represents an attractive alternative to autofluorescence because of enhanced fluorescence emission and potential selectivity of the fluorophore for neoplastic tissue. The most commonly studied agents have been photosensitizers used in photodynamic therapy, such as porfimer sodium and 5-aminolevulinic acid (5-ALA). The latter is a precursor molecule, which induces the production of an endogenous fluorophore, protoporphyrin IX (PpIX). Fluorescence signal detection is facilitated, since optimal excitation and emission wavelengths of these drugs are known a priori. However, for most agents, uncertainty exists regarding the optimal drug dose, route of administration, and/or time delay to detection. Moreover, the application of drug-enhanced fluorescence detection at the time of endoscopy has been limited by several factors, including variable drug uptake and distribution in neoplastic tissue, adverse effects, costs, and lack of regulatory approval for this purpose.

Table 1
Endogenous tissue fluorophores

Fluorophores	Origins	Optimal Excitation Wavelength (nm)	Peak Fluorescence Emission (nm)
Tryptophan	Protein	280	350
Tyrosine		275	300
Phenylalanine		260	280
Collagen	Connective tissue	330	390
Elastin		360	410
NADH	Respiratory chain	340	450
Flavins		450	520
Porphyrins	Heme biosynthesis by-products; bacterial fauna	400–450	635, 690

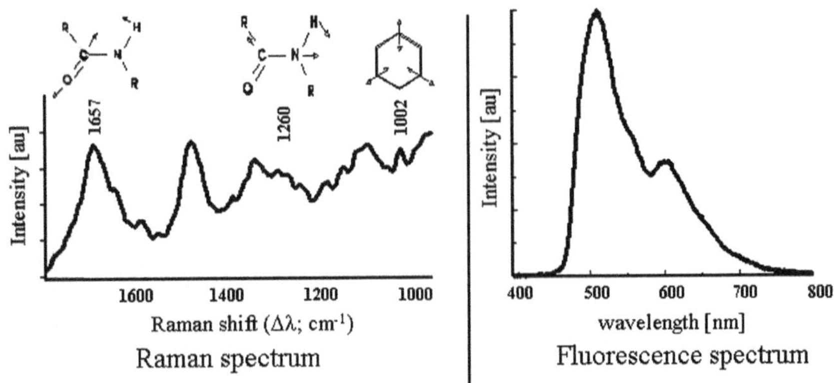

Fig. 2. Fluorescence vs Raman spectra of normal esophagus. Raman spectral features are more detailed, which may translate into more accurate tissue diagnosis.

Endoscopic Applications

Evaluation of the diagnostic performance of point fluorescence spectroscopy in the GI tract is limited to feasibility studies, as summarized in **Tables 2** and **3**.[4–14,16–20] Moreover, there is heterogeneity in experimental design, sample size, wavelength selection, and/or methods of spectral analysis in several fluorescence studies published to date. Consequently, a wide range of diagnostic sensitivities and specificities have been reported for the differentiation of Barrett's epithelia and colon polyps. In general, the diagnostic sensitivity of autofluorescence spectroscopy is good to excellent for lesion differentiation, particularly for colon polyps. False positives occur in the setting of inflammatory or reactive changes, thereby limiting diagnostic specificity. The use of

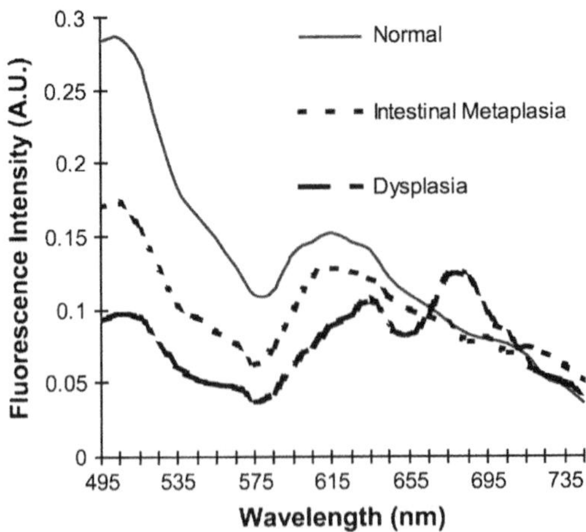

Fig. 3. Mean normalized fluorescence emission spectra of normal squamous esophagus, nondysplastic Barrett's esophagus, and dysplastic Barrett's esophagus following 437-nm excitation. The spectral dip at about 580 nm is attributed to hemoglobin absorption. (*From* Wong Kee Song LM, Marcon NE. Novel optical diagnostic techniques for the recognition of metaplasia and dysplasia. In: Sharma P, Sampliner RE, editors. Barrett's esophagus and esophageal adenocarcinoma. Boston: Blackwell Science; 2001. p. 123–36; with permission.)

drug-enhanced fluorescence spectroscopy in the GI tract is evolving, but existing studies have yet to demonstrate a significant diagnostic advantage over autofluorescence.[12–14]

Most in vivo studies to date have reported the use of steady-state fluorescence measurements. Time-resolved autofluorescence spectroscopy is an alternative approach in which time-resolved fluorescence spectra represent, at a given emission wavelength, the decay of fluorescence intensity as a function of time after a brief pulse of excitation light (~10 ns). In one study, the fluorescence time decay of colonic adenomas was found to be shorter than that of nonadenomatous polyps, yielding a sensitivity of 85% and a specificity of 91% for polyp differentiation.[19] Further studies are needed to validate the diagnostic accuracy of this technique in the GI tract.

Future Prospects

Advances in fluorescence detection rest on the development of "contrast agents" that are highly selective for markers of neoplasia. In the case of fluorescence contrast agents, the challenges include identifying suitable biomarkers of disease against which to target the fluorophores and selecting the optimum fluorophores. The conjugation of fluorescent organic dyes or nanoparticles (eg, semiconductor quantum dots) to monoclonal antibodies, enzymes, or other dysplasia-/tumor-targeting moieties holds significant promise in improving fluorescence detection or differentiation of lesions with high diagnostic accuracy from either a spectroscopic or imaging approach.[22]

RAMAN SPECTROSCOPY

Principles

Raman scattering consists of slight shifts in frequency (or wavelength) of scattered light relative to the incident light due to exchange of energy between light photons and molecular structures of tissue. These wavelength shifts (expressed in wave numbers, cm^{-1}) correspond to specific vibrations or rotations of particular molecular bonds (see **Fig. 2**). Molecular vibrations originating from proteins, lipids, or nucleic acids all exhibit distinct Raman signatures. For example, the peak at 1002 cm^{-1} in **Fig. 2** corresponds to the "in and out" vibrations of phenyl rings of aromatic amino acids. Relative to fluorescence, Raman signals are spectrally detailed with many peaks and bands, which may translate into more accurate tissue diagnosis or discrimination. The Raman phenomenon, however, is a rare event, since only a small fraction of light undergoes Raman (inelastic) scattering following light interaction with tissue molecules. Almost all of the light that is scattered by tissue is of the same wavelength as the incident light (elastic scattering).

Raman scattering, therefore, is more difficult to measure, since the signal is much weaker relative to fluorescence or elastic scattering. Moreover, the application of Raman spectroscopy using fiber-optic probes at the time of endoscopy has been technically challenging due to spectral "contamination" from background tissue fluorescence and fluorescence and Raman signals generated in the fiber-optic materials. Sophisticated signal processing/analysis and recent technological advances in high-throughput spectrographs, high-sensitivity, near-infrared detectors, and filtered fiber-optic probes have enabled near-infrared Raman spectroscopy instruments to be developed for endoscopic use.[15,21,23,24]

Although Raman scattering can be induced by ultraviolet, visible, or near-infrared light, the light source selected for endoscopic applications is a near-infrared laser (eg, 785 nm), which minimizes excitation of interfering tissue autofluorescence while

Table 2
Selected in vivo studies of fluorescence and Raman spectroscopy in the esophagus

Authors	Technique	λ_{exc} (nm)	λ_{em} (nm)	Patients (n)	Spectra/ Tissue (n)	Diagnostic Algorithm	Findings/ Comments
Panjehpour et al[4] (1995)	AFS	410	430–716	32	123 normal 36 SCC and ACA	LDA	Sn 100% and Sp 98% for SCC/ ACA vs normal
Vo-Dinh et al[5] (1995)	AFS	410	430–720	48	>200 normal and SCC/ACA spectra	DNF	>98% accuracy
Panjehpour et al[6] (1996)	AFS	410	430–716	36	216 NDB 36 LGD 46 focal HGD 10 diffuse HGD	$DNF_{480\ nm}$ and $DNF_{660\ nm}$	Sn 100% and Sp 70% for HGD vs rest. Technique insensitive at detecting LGD
Bourg-Heckly et al[7] (2000)	AFS	330	350–650	24	66 normal 116 NDB 11 dysplastic 25 SCC and ACA	$I_{390\ nm}/I_{550\ nm}$	Sn 86% and Sp 95% for HGD/ ACA/SCC vs. normal/NDB
Wang et al[8] (2001)	AFS	337	350–800	87	266 NDB 46 LGD 14 HGD	Proprietary algorithm	Sn 95% and Sp 80% for HGD vs NDB/LGD
Georgakoudi et al[9] (2001)	AFS	11 λ_{exc} (between 337 and 620)	350–750	18	26 NDB 7 LGD 7 HGD	PCA and LRA	Sn 100% and Sp 97% for HGD vs NDB/LGD Sn 79% and Sp 88% for LGD/HGD vs NDB
Mayinger et al[10] (2001)	AFS	375–478	478–700	13	57 normal 55 SCC 17 ACA	$I_{500–549\ nm}/I_{657–700\ nm}$	Sn 97% and Sp 95% for SCC/ACA vs normal

Pfefer et al[11] (2003)	AFS	337 and 400	—	37	—	LDA	Sn 74% and Sp 67%–85% for HGD; steady-state measurements more effective than time-resolved
Von Holstein et al[12] (1996)	DFS (porfimer sodium)	405	450–750	5	48 normal/NDB 17 ACA	$I_{630\ nm}/I_{500\ nm}$	Sn 88% and Sp 94% for ACA vs normal/NDB
Brand et al[13] (2002)	DFS (5-ALA)	400	—	20	97 total 13 HGD	Quantitative normalized PpIX fluorescence intensity peak @ 635 nm	Sn 77% and Sp 71% for HGD
Ortner et al[14] (2003)	DFS (5-ALA)	505	5-ALA-induced PpIX fluorescence	53	141 total 9 HGD/ACA	PpIX red fluorescence	Sn 76% and Sp 63% for detecting LGD/HGD/ACA vs NDB
Wong Kee Song et al[15] (2005)	RS	785	900–1800 cm^{-1}	65	112 NDB 54 LGD 26 HGD/ACA	LDA	Sn 88% and Sp 89% for HGD/ACA vs NDB/LGD

Abbreviations: ACA, adenocarcinoma in Barrett's esophagus; AFS, autofluorescence spectroscopy; 5-ALA, 5-aminolevulinic acid; DFS, drug-enhanced fluorescence spectroscopy; DNF, differential normalized fluorescence; HGD, high-grade dysplasia; I, fluorescence intensity; LDA, linear discriminant analysis; LGD, low-grade dysplasia; LRA, logistic regression analysis; NDB, non-dysplastic Barrett; PCA, principal component analysis; PpIX, protoporphyrin IX; RS, Raman spectroscopy; SCC, squamous cell cancer; Sn, sensitivity; Sp, specificity; λ_{exc}, excitation wavelength(s); λ_{em}, emission wavelengths.

Table 3
Selected in vivo studies of fluorescence and Raman spectroscopy in the colon

Authors	Technique	λ_{exc} (nm)	Patients (n)	Spectra/Tissue (n)	Diagnostic Algorithm	Findings/Comments
Cothren et al[16] (1990)	AFS	370	20	31 Adenomas 4 hyperplastic 32 normal	$I_{460\ nm}$ vs $I_{680\ nm}$ scatter plot	Sn 100% and Sp 97% for adenomas
Cothren et al[17] (1996)	AFS	370	57	29 Adenomas 59 normal and hyperplastic	Probability-based algorithm (I_{460} and I_{680}/I_{600})	Sn 90% and Sp 95% for adenomas
Shomacker et al[18] (1992)	AFS	337	49	49 Adenomas 35 hyperplastic	Linear regression analysis	Sn 86% and Sp 80% for adenomas
Mycek et al[19] (1998)	AFS	337	17	13 Adenomas 11 nonadenomas	Decay time Scatter plot	Sn 85% and Sp 91% for adenomas
Mayinger B[20] (2003)	AFS	375–478	23	72 Cancer 89 adenomas 13 hyperplastic 137 normal	Intensity ratio ($I_{500\text{-}549\ nm}/I_{657\text{-}700\ nm}$)	Sn 96% and Sp 93% for rectal cancer; Sn 98% and Sp 89% for adenomas
Molckovsky A[21] (2003)	RS	785	8	10 Adenomas 9 hyperplastic	PCA, LDA	Sn 100% and Sp 89% for adenomas

Abbreviations: AFS, autofluorescence spectroscopy; HGD, high-grade dysplasia; I, fluorescence intensity; LDA, linear discriminant analysis; PCA, principal component analysis; RS, Raman spectroscopy; Sn, sensitivity; Sp, specificity; λ_{exc}, excitation wavelength(s).

generating Raman signals sensitive enough to be detected by available charge-coupled device cameras. Even though the instrumentation design is similar (see **Fig. 1**), Raman technology is more expensive than fluorescence, because more complex spectroscopic components and specialized fiber-optic probes are required to detect the weak Raman signal of the tissue. Moreover, complex, multivariate statistical techniques are required for spectral analysis to sort out the subtle yet potentially discriminatory spectral differences observed between tissue types (**Fig. 4**).

Endoscopic Applications

The diagnostic potential of near-infrared Raman spectroscopy for lesion differentiation at the time of endoscopy is promising. In a feasibility study involving 65 patients with Barrett's esophagus, Raman spectroscopy identified lesions containing high-grade dysplasia or early cancer with an overall diagnostic accuracy of 89%.[15] In a small proof-of-concept study, Raman spectroscopy distinguished adenomas (n = 10) from hyperplastic polyps (n = 9) with 100% sensitivity, 89% specificity, and 95% accuracy.[21] In an ex vivo study, Raman spectroscopy yielded 95% sensitivity and 91% specificity for distinguishing gastric dysplasia from normal gastric tissue.[25]

Future Prospects

Future Raman developments may involve the use of alternative spectral ranges that may overcome some of the current technical limitations[26] and methods that can markedly increase the signal strength of Raman spectroscopy. For the latter, options include the use of Coherent Anti-Stokes Raman scattering, using "stimulated" rather than spontaneous inelastic scattering, and the use of surface-enhanced Raman spectroscopy in which the Raman signal is amplified in close proximity to metal nanoparticles. Thus, the nanoparticles can serve as either "reporters" or "amplifiers" of the

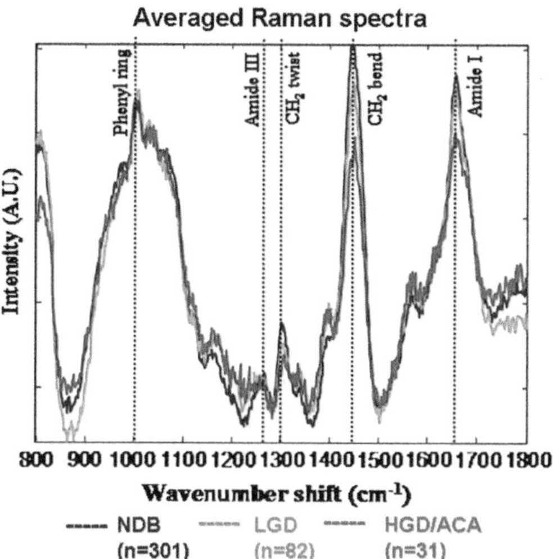

Fig. 4. Average in vivo Raman spectra of nondysplastic Barrett's tissue sites (NDB, n = 301), low-grade dysplasia (LGD, n = 82), and high-grade dysplasia/early adenocarcinoma (HGD/ACA, n = 31) from 65 patients with Barrett's esophagus. Typical tissue Raman peaks are labeled. Subtle but potentially discriminatory spectral differences are present throughout, requiring multivariate techniques for tissue classification (see text).

Raman information. These options also open the potential for in vivo endoscopic Raman imaging, which is currently not feasible with existing techniques.

SUMMARY

Several proof-of-concept studies have demonstrated the potential of fluorescence and Raman spectroscopy for lesion diagnosis or differentiation in the GI tract. It is anticipated that future technological developments will further improve the diagnostic efficiency of these techniques and move these modalities from the proof-of-concept stage to clinically useful and viable devices.

REFERENCES

1. Wong Kee Song LM, Wilson BC. Endoscopic detection of early upper GI cancers. Best Pract Res Clin Gastroenterol 2005;19(6):833–56.
2. DaCosta RS, Wilson BC, Marcon NE. Optical techniques for the endoscopic detection of dysplastic colonic lesions. Curr Opin Gastroenterol 2005;21(1):70–9.
3. Georgakoudi I, Jacobson BC, Muller MG, et al. NAD(P)H and collagen as in vivo quantitative fluorescent biomarkers of epithelial precancerous changes. Cancer Res 2002;62(3):682–7.
4. Panjehpour M, Overholt BF, Schmidhammer JL, et al. Spectroscopic diagnosis of esophageal cancer: new classification model, improved measurement system. Gastrointest Endosc 1995;41(6):577–81.
5. Vo-Dinh T, Panjehpour M, Overholt BF, et al. In vivo cancer diagnosis of the esophagus using differential normalized fluorescence (DNF) indices. Lasers Surg Med 1995;16(1):41–7.
6. Panjehpour M, Overholt BF, Vo-Dinh T, et al. Endoscopic fluorescence detection of high-grade dysplasia in Barrett's esophagus. Gastroenterology 1996;111(1):93–101.
7. Bourg-Heckly G, Blais J, Padilla JJ, et al. Endoscopic ultraviolet-induced autofluorescence spectroscopy of the esophagus: tissue characterization and potential for early cancer diagnosis. Endoscopy 2000;32(10):756–65.
8. Wang KK, Buttar NS, Wong Kee Song LM, et al. The use of an optical biopsy system in Barrett's esophagus [abstract]. Gastroenterology 2001;120:A2112.
9. Georgakoudi I, Jacobson BC, Van Dam J, et al. Fluorescence, reflectance, and light-scattering spectroscopy for evaluating dysplasia in patients with Barrett's esophagus. Gastroenterology 2001;120(7):1620–9.
10. Mayinger B, Horner P, Jordan M, et al. Light-induced autofluorescence spectroscopy for the endoscopic detection of esophageal cancer. Gastrointest Endosc 2001;54(2):195–201.
11. Pfefer TJ, Paithankar DY, Poneros JM, et al. Temporally and spectrally resolved fluorescence spectroscopy for the detection of high grade dysplasia in Barrett's esophagus. Lasers Surg Med 2003;32(1):10–6.
12. Von Holstein CS, Nilsson AMK, Andersson-Engels S, et al. Detection of adenocarcinoma in Barrett's oesophagus by means of laser induced fluorescence. Gut 1996;39(5):711–6.
13. Brand S, Wang TD, Schomacker KT, et al. Detection of high-grade dysplasia in Barrett's esophagus by spectroscopy measurement of 5-aminolevulinic acid-induced protoporphyrin IX fluorescence. Gastrointest Endosc 2002;56(4):479–87.
14. Ortner MA, Ebert B, Hein E, et al. Time gated fluorescence spectroscopy in Barrett's oesophagus. Gut 2003;52(1):28–33.

15. Wong Kee Song LM, Molckovsky A, Wang KK, et al. Diagnostic potential of Raman spectroscopy in Barrett's esophagus. Proc Soc Photo Opt Instrum Eng 2005;5692: 140–6.
16. Cothren RM, Richards-Kortum R, Sivak MV Jr, et al. Gastrointestinal tissue diagnosis by laser-induced fluorescence spectroscopy at endoscopy. Gastrointest Endosc 1990;36(2):105–11.
17. Cothren RM, Sivak MV Jr, Van Dam J, et al. Detection of dysplasia at colonoscopy using laser-induced fluorescence: a blinded study. Gastrointest Endosc 1996; 44(2):168–76.
18. Schomacker KT, Frisoli JK, Compton CC, et al. Ultraviolet laser-induced fluorescence of colonic polyps. Gastroenterology 1992;102(4 Pt 1):1155–60.
19. Mycek MA, Schomacker KT, Nishioka NS. Colonic polyp differentiation using time-resolved autofluorescence spectroscopy. Gastrointest Endosc 1998;48(4): 390–4.
20. Mayinger B, Jordan M, Horner P, et al. Endoscopic light-induced autofluorescence spectroscopy for the diagnosis of colorectal cancer and adenoma. J Photochem Photobiol B 2003;70(1):13–20.
21. Molckovsky A, Wong Kee Song LM, Shim MG, et al. Diagnostic potential of near-infrared Raman spectroscopy in the colon: differentiating adenomatous from hyperplastic polyps. Gastrointest Endosc 2003;57(3):396–402.
22. Dacosta RS, Wilson BC, Marcon NE. Fluorescence and spectral imaging. ScientificWorldJournal 2007;21(7):2046–71.
23. Choo-Smith LP, Edwards HG, Endtz HP, et al. Medical applications of Raman spectroscopy: from proof of principle to clinical implementation. Biopolymers 2002;67(1):1–9.
24. Shim MG, Wong Kee Song LM, Marcon NE, et al. In vivo near-infrared Raman spectroscopy: demonstration of feasibility during clinical gastrointestinal endoscopy. Photochem Photobiol 2000;72(1):146–50.
25. Teh SK, Zheng W, Ho KY, et al. Diagnostic potential of near-infrared Raman spectroscopy in the stomach: differentiating dysplasia from normal tissue. Br J Cancer 2008;98(2):457–65.
26. Santos LF, Wolthuis R, Koljenović S, et al. Fiber-optic probes for in vivo Raman spectroscopy in the high-wave number region. Anal Chem 2005; 77(20):6747–52.

Reflectance Spectroscopy

Michael B. Wallace, MD, MPH[a,*], Adam Wax, PhD[b], David N. Roberts, MD[c], Robert N. Graf, PhD[b]

KEYWORDS

• Spectroscopy • Endoscopy • Light scattering • Dysplasia
• Barret's esophagus • Colotis • Colorectal polyps

Reflectance spectroscopy is an emerging technology among the new optically based endoscopic techniques. Providing a rapid and safe evaluation of tissue for dysplasia and ischemia without excision, it overcomes many limitations in histopathologic processing and diagnosis. Reflectance spectroscopy is a form of point-probe technology that has the advantages of ease of passage through the accessory channel of a standard diagnostic endoscope and predictable geometry between fibers that provide the light source and those that deliver collected light to the detector. It quantitatively measures the color and intensity of reflected light. Unlike autofluorescence spectroscopy, the reflected light maintains the same wavelength, although different wavelengths are absorbed and reflected to different degrees.

A standard example is oxygenated hemoglobin, which, when illuminated with white light, absorbs much of the blue light and reflects back the red light, giving its characteristic color. Deoxygenated hemoglobin absorbs a higher degree of red light, appearing bluer when illuminated with white light. Reflectance spectroscopy provides information about tissue hemoglobin concentrations and oxygenation status. With the inherent property of malignant tissue to promote angiogenesis, reflectance spectroscopy may be capable of detecting neoplastic tissue based on hemoglobin absorption parameters.

Light-scattering spectroscopy (LSS) is a form of reflectance spectroscopy, which uses the properties of elastic scattering inherent to structures within the tissues. It measures the extent to which the angular paths of light are altered by structures such as nuclei, mitochondria, and collagen networks. Described herein, further advancements of these principles have provided other potential tools for diagnostic purposes.

This work was supported by Grant R33-CA109907 from the National Cancer Institute.
[a] Division of Gastroenterology, Mayo Clinic, 4500 San Pablo Road, Jacksonville, FL, USA
[b] Department of Biomedical Engineering, Duke University, Durham, NC 27708, USA
[c] Digestive Diseases Section, University of Oklahoma, 920 Stanton L Young Boulevard, WP 1360, Oklahoma City, OK 73013, USA
* Corresponding author.
E-mail address: wallace.michael@mayo.edu (M.B. Wallace).

Gastrointest Endoscopy Clin N Am 19 (2009) 233–242
doi:10.1016/j.giec.2009.02.008 **giendo.theclinics.com**
1052-5157/09/$ – see front matter

Light reflected from tissue is modified by the processes of absorption and scattering (**Fig. 1**). Absorption of light in the body occurs at specific wavelengths, which depend on the biochemical makeup of the probed tissue. In comparison, light scattering produces changes in the trajectory of incident light and affects all wavelengths across the visible spectrum to varying degrees. Light scattering in tissue is determined by the micron-scale morphology of the probed sample. The interplay of these two processes, absorption and scattering, provides access to a rich source of information for assessing the health status of tissues. By examining the wavelength of reflected light, information about tissue absorption can be obtained. Light scattering, on the other hand, provides information about the way in which photons propagate through tissues, providing structural knowledge of the morphology within. Like absorption, scattering information can be obtained by examining the spectral dependence of detected light. After accounting for absorption, the wavelength-specific intensities of scattered light, which contain unique scattering signatures, can be analyzed. Quantitative morphologic information about the probed tissue can be obtained through more sophisticated analysis of the angular, polarization, and wavelength dependence of the scattered light.

Absorption of light occurs when the energy of a photon is absorbed and converted to heat energy. Tissue absorption is characterized using the Beer-Lambert law of exponential attenuation with photon path length. The absorption coefficient, μa, is generally wavelength dependent for biochemicals of interest. The absorption coefficient depends on the concentration and molar absorptivity of biochemicals present in the tissue. The most common tissue absorber is hemoglobin, which has a characteristic absorption spectrum. Oxygenated and deoxygenated hemoglobin preferentially absorb light of different wavelengths, as evidenced by the more reddish color of oxygenated blood and the more bluish color of deoxygenated blood. The extent of absorption by each type of hemoglobin provides information about their relative concentrations and indirectly provides information about the vascularity and metabolic status of tissue. This is the principal behind optical pulse oximeters, which perform an extremely simplistic form of reflectance spectroscopy. Hemoglobin absorption can be used as an indicator for many disease states. For example,

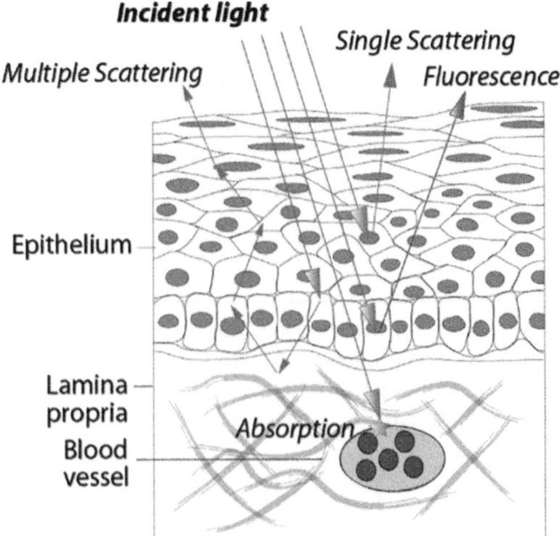

Fig. 1. Interactions between light and tissue include single or multiple scattering, absorption, or fluorescence.

malignant and premalignant gastrointestinal (GI) tissues tend to be more vascular (with higher concentrations of hemoglobin) and also more metabolically active (and thus higher ratios of deoxy:oxyhemoglobin). Tissue that is also poorly perfused, such as in chronic intestinal ischemia, can also be detected using reflectance spectroscopy, in this case with lower levels of hemoglobin and higher ratios of deoxy:oxyhemoglobin.

LSS is a type of reflectance spectroscopy that determines tissue structures by examining elastic scattering. Elastic light scattering is a process in which the illumination light does not undergo a shift in wavelength during the scattering event. Each wavelength of the illumination light is scattered to a different degree by dense structures in the tissue such as nuclei. A portion of the light incident on the tissue is backscattered, or scattered directly in the backward direction, and can be collected by the fiber optic probe that delivered the light to the tissue or a distinct collection optical fiber. Since no energy is lost during these scattering events, and therefore no wavelength shift occurs, this type of spectroscopy is termed "elastic." By analyzing the varying degree to which individual wavelengths are backscattered across a spectral range, it is possible to determine the size, number, and optical density of the dense structures within a tissue. This light scattering information can be used to detect developing abnormalities in a tissue. For example, neoplastic tissue, which is characterized by enlarged nuclei, can be accurately detected at its earliest stages by elastic scattering spectroscopy.

EQUIPMENT FOR MEASURING REFLECTANCE

A key advantage of using reflectance spectroscopy as a method for diagnosing tissue health is the wide availability and ease of use of the optical instrumentation. The telecom boom of the late 1990s led to the availability of many off-the-shelf fiber optic components, which have been adapted for biomedical spectroscopy by the new field of biophotonics. Further advances in computing power, data transfer, and optical instrumentation have further fueled advances in this field. Reflectance spectroscopy systems for biomedical applications contain three key components: a light source, a fiber optic probe, and a spectrometer. The particular specifications chosen for of each of these components, along with the methods of analyzing the collected data, suit particular reflectance spectroscopy systems in certain clinical applications.

The light source of a reflectance spectroscopy system is selected primarily based on its brightness and wavelength range. The brightness, or power output, of a light source must be high enough so that the reflected signal is sufficiently stronger than the background noise signal such that high-fidelity measurements can be made on reasonable time scales. When performing reflectance spectroscopy in vivo, the power of the light incident on tissue must also conform to the maximum power level allowable by American National Standards Institute standards so as not to damage the tissue. Coherent light sources, such as lasers and superluminescent diodes, typically illuminate tissue with significantly higher power than white-light arc lamp sources, especially when delivered through optical fibers. Although increased brightness offers the potential of a better signal-to-noise ratio, power levels must be carefully measured to prevent thermally damaging the probed tissue.

The wavelength range of a given light source is also typically tailored to a particular application. Some light sources, such as white-light arc lamps, span the entire visible spectrum and extend into the ultraviolet and near-infrared ranges but may present undesirable features, such as sharp spectral peaks and substantial infrared components, which can heat the tissue. Coherent light sources, however, span a smaller range from a single wavelength up to several 10s of nanometers. In the case of a small wavelength range, a light source whose illumination includes the most diagnostically relevant wavelengths for a particular application should be selected. For broadband light sources, it is important to ensure that all the included wavelength components are transmitted satisfactorily through the optical system, avoiding dispersion effects.

The second major component of a reflectance spectroscopy system is a fiber optic probe. The fiber probe both delivers excitation light to the tissue of interest and collects the reflected signal. The use of thin, flexible fiber optics allows light to be delivered to almost any hollow organ of the body. The probes are typically designed to work seamlessly with the auxiliary port of standard endoscopes. The specific geometry and design of the probe can be tailored to meet the specific needs of the application. For example, the degree of tissue penetration and the angle of interface with tissue can be customized by refining the fiber probe geometry. Illumination and signal collection can be accomplished with a single fiber or with a series of fibers grouped in a bundle depending on the intended application.

The spectrometer is the final major component of a reflectance spectroscopy system. Spectrometers split the detected signal into individual wavelength components and detect their respective intensities using a CCD chip or another multichannel detector. The size and design of a spectrometer dictate the spectral resolution and the range of detectible wavelengths. These specifications have a trade-off relationship, that is, an increase in spectral resolution results in a decrease in wavelength range and vice versa. Modern spectrometers are available in compact footprints that are ideal for clinical applications. Most systems interface with computers via USB, which permit high-speed acquisition control and transfer of data. Commercial spectrometers can be controlled via basic, easy-to-use commercial software packages or via customized software, which allows for more sophisticated data analysis that can often be performed in real or near real-time.

Although the traditional instrument used in reflectance spectroscopy is the spectrometer, advances in spectroscopic techniques have enabled better tissue characterization. We discuss recent developments in optical methods and advantages of novel fiber probe geometries as they relate to clinical application. A significant influence on the usefulness of reflected light for tissue diagnosis is the method of analysis. Although empiric methods can be used to diagnose diseased tissues, advances in physical modeling of the interaction between light and tissues have lead to improved methods for tissue analysis. By linking spectral features to specific tissue characteristics, novel analysis models have provided more detailed information on tissue composition. We discuss how the use of advanced physical models can provide superior diagnostic capability.

CLINICAL APPLICATIONS

Reflectance spectroscopy techniques have shown important applications in key clinical settings, including GI ischemia, dysplasia, and neoplasia. Although in infancy of use, these techniques have shown tremendous potential in early studies for widespread application.

Multiple forms of radiographic imaging are available to evaluate for mesenteric ischemia. Acute mesenteric ischemia is often clinically diagnosed early on based on clinical history and symptomatic presentation. On the other hand, chronic mesenteric ischemia can be much more difficult to diagnose, with some patients lacking classic symptoms and others presenting with nonspecific abdominal pain. Mesenteric angiography, duplex ultrasonography, computerized tomographic angiography, and magnetic resonance angiography all provide excellent forms to evaluate for stenotic lesions to account for symptoms. An endoscopic diagnostic method, however, is potentially advantageous for many patients in that endoscopic evaluation is often performed early on in the diagnostic workup for abdominal pain. Quantitative measurements of mucosal capillary hemoglobin oxygen saturation would also provide an objective, reproducible means to assess the degree of ischemia before and after any intervention.

A fiberoptic, catheter-based, visible light spectroscopy oximeter was developed for the purpose of continuously measuring mucosal tissue oxygen saturation and has been evaluated for proof of concept in colonic mucosa before and after submucosal epinephrine injection and strangulation of polyp stalks by endoloop in normal volunteers. Oxygen saturations at baseline, before manipulation, were between 60% and 80%. When altered by injection or strangulation, desaturations of the mucosal stalk occurred rapidly down to 18% to 36%.[1]

This was further demonstrated in three patients with abdominal pain, weight loss, and medical risk factors for chronic mesenteric ischemia. Baseline oximetry measurements were obtained from 25 to 30 healthy controls, with normal mucosa in the esophagus, stomach, duodenum/jejunum, and colon/rectum. The 3 patients evaluated had clear evidence of mucosal abnormalities ranging from cyanotic, friable, and erythematous to diffuse erosions and ulcerations. A statistically significant difference in tissue saturation was demonstrated in different segments of the small bowel between the healthy patients and the three cases before intervention ($P = .003$). One patient had an increase in proximal jejunum saturation from 30% to 60% after vascular intervention. Another had dramatic improvement in the duodenum (19% to 51%) and proximal jejunum (42% to 56%) following intervention. The third had changes from 16% to 59% in the proximal jejunum, and mid-duodenal measurements improved from 45% to 55% with resolution of gastric ulcers and mottling within 3 days. Aside from a small patient study size, the technique has limitations in potential sampling error, difficulty reaching the mucosal area of injury, and the likelihood that patients with milder ischemic changes would expectantly have oximetry values much closer to normal. This technique does have other potential applications, however, in the evaluation of intestinal ischemia at surgical anastomoses and postoperative strictures.[2]

LSS has been shown for many years to have potential use in the detection of dysplasia and carcinoma in situ in a variety of organ systems and epithelial cell types, including transitional cell epithelium of the bladder, squamous lining of the oral cavity, and columnar cells of the colon and Barrett's esophagus. The nuclear-size distribution and refractive index were determined, allowing for quantification of nuclear enlargement, crowding, and hyperchromasia.[3]

In evaluation of patients with Barrett's esophagus, 13 consecutive patients were analyzed endoscopically with the use of LSS. White light spectroscopy was used to assess the size distribution of cell nuclei. These data were extrapolated to determine the percentage of enlarged nuclei and degree of nuclear crowding. Dysplasia was assigned if more than 30% of the nuclei exceeded 10 μm and there was histologic agreement with four blinded pathologists. The sensitivity and specificity for LSS in detecting either high-grade dysplasia (HGD) or low-grade dysplasia (LGD) were 90% and 90%, respectively. All HGD samples were properly characterized as such by LSS, and 87% of LGD lesions classified correctly.[4]

In a study of the rat esophagus carcinogenesis model, the angle-resolved low coherence interferometry (a/LCI) light scattering technique was applied to detect nuclear morphology changes due to neoplastic transformation (**Fig. 2**). In this approach, the unique coherence gating capability of this technique was used to isolate light scattered exclusively from the basal layer of the epithelium. The angular

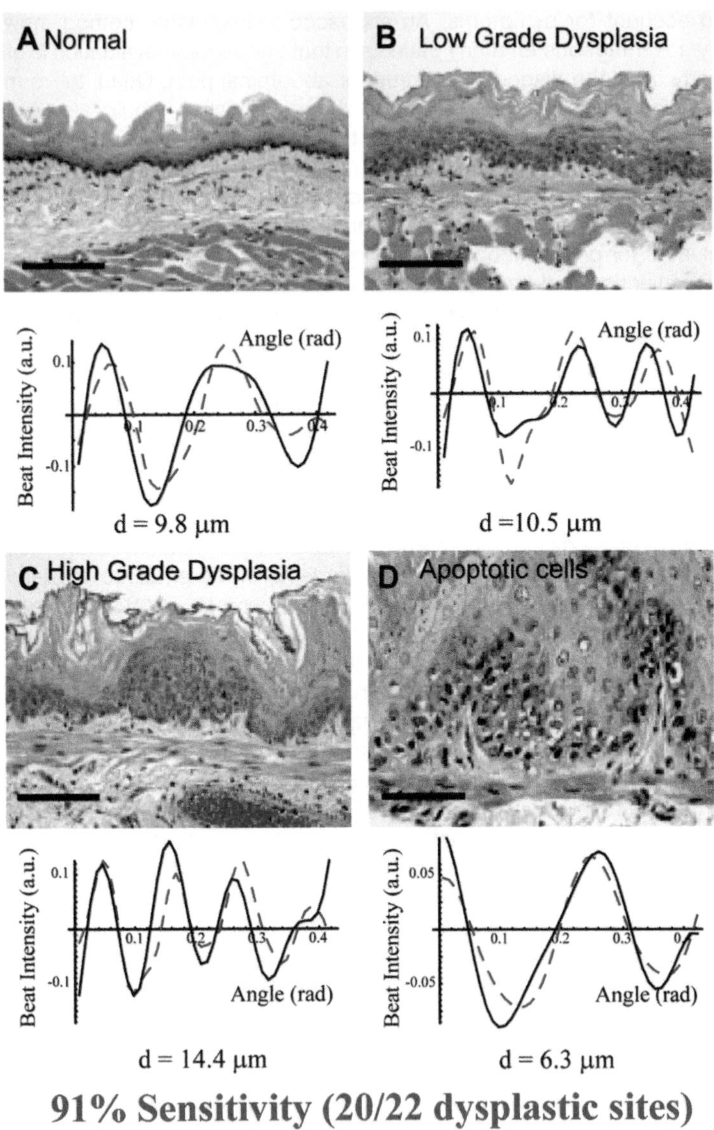

Fig. 2. (*A, B*) Angle-resolved low coherence interferometry (a/LCI) in a rat esophagus model of colon carcinogenesis shows increasing hemoglobin detected by 4D-ELF prior to the development of aberrant crypt foci.

distribution of scattered light was used to detect changes in the average size of the cell nuclei in response to treatment with the carcinogen NMBA (*N*-nitrosomethylbenzylamine). Logistic regression revealed that nucleus size was a powerful indicator of precancerous lesions, yielding 80% sensitivity and 100% specificity.[5] Significantly, this study also revealed chemopreventive action by detecting contracted cell nuclei identified as apoptotic. A follow-up study using a/LCI employed the decision line from the first study to prospectively grade tissue samples from this animal model at multiple time points. The technique was found to have high sensitivity (91%) and specificity (97%) for detecting precancerous lesions in this model.[6]

In analyzing models of colon carcinogenesis, 4-dimensional elastic light scattering fingerprinting (4D-ELF), a type of LSS was applied to examine the colonic mucosa from rats, which were induced toward dysplastic transformation using the carcinogen azoxymethane (AOM). The light scattering data were analyzed using 4D-ELF to determine if preneoplastic changes could be detected. About 48 rats were randomized to weekly injections of saline or AOM for two doses. The animals were harvested from 2 to 20 weeks after the second injection for colon mucosal evaluation. A subset of rat colons was further assessed for aberrant crypt foci (ACF). Induction of ACF by AOM became apparent within 4 to 6 weeks of the second injection; ACF were predominantly located in the distal colon and continued to increase over time. Notably, even before the development of ACF, at 2-week analysis, significant changes were present in the 4D-ELF fingerprint signatures (**Fig. 3**). These microarchitectural abnormalities are

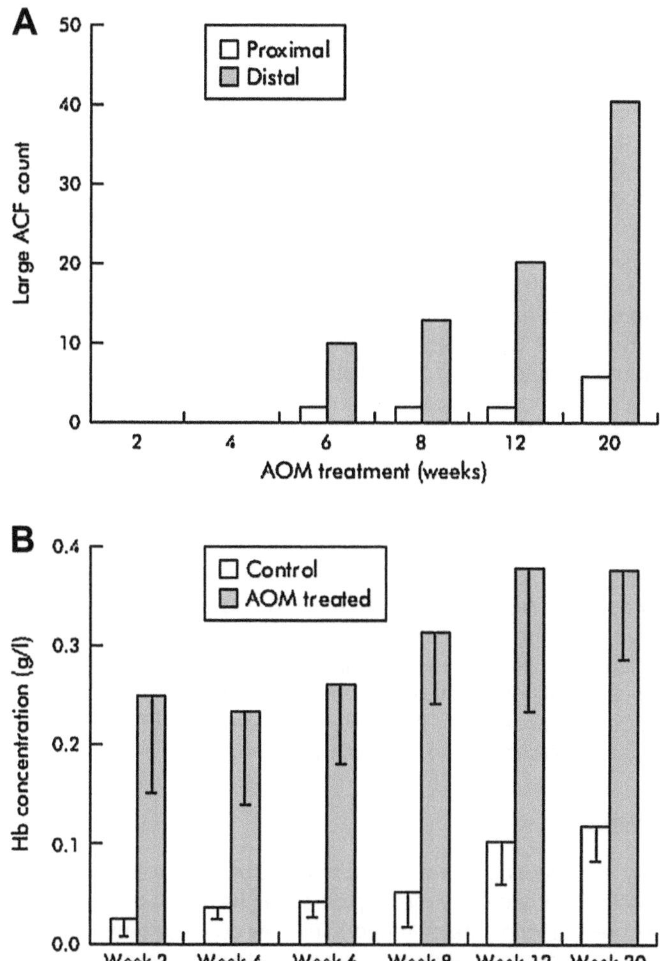

Fig. 3. (*A, B*) 4-dimentional light scattering fingerprinting (4D-ELF) in a rat model of colon carcinogenesis shows increasing hemoglobin detected by 4D-ELF prior to the development of aberrant crypt foci.

important in carcinogenesis, as they correlate temporally and spatially with subsequent ACF. These detectable alterations in 4D-ELF signatures suggest the presence of a field effect, a feature strongly desirable in early carcinoma detection.[7]

4D-ELF was further used to evaluate the superficial blood content in colonic mucosa of Fischer rats induced toward neoplastic changes with AOM. The depth of focused analysis involved the pericryptal capillary plexus and demonstrated significant, reproducible differences between control and preneoplastic mucosa. In addition, multiple intestinal neoplasia mice were evaluated with 4D-ELF for red blood cell content in the small bowel and colonic mucosa. These mice possess a germline mutation in the APC tumor suppressor gene, which results in small-bowel polyps and neoplasia. As expected, before neoplastic transformation, there was a marked fingerprinting change in the small intestine but not in the colonic mucosa. Subsequently, a pilot study in the normal-appearing mucosa of the transverse colon in 37 patients undergoing routine colonoscopy was performed to evaluate for early increase in blood supply. 4D-ELF analysis of the mucosa revealed a three-fold increased in superficial blood in patients with advanced adenomas, defined as an adenoma greater than or equal to 1 cm, with HGD or a greater than 25% villous component. Importantly, none of the high-grade lesions was present in the transverse colon but in the cecum, rectum, and sigmoid colon.[8] Clearly, further studies need to be performed with a larger patient cohort to evaluate if these findings are reproducible to determine if this spectroscopic technique would benefit patients widespread in screening protocols for colon carcinoma.

In the arena of pancreatic adenocarcinoma, 4D-ELF and low-coherence enhanced backscattering (LEBS) technologies have been recently used to evaluate normal-appearing periampullary duodenal wall biopsies in 19 patients with pancreatic cancer compared with 32 healthy controls. These samples were taken between 1 and 3 cm from the ampulla and evaluated histologically by a pathologist to confirm that no dysplasia or neoplasia was present in the tissue specimen. In addition, biopsies were taken in the stomach and 10 cm distal to the ampulla in nine patients from the malignant cohort and four of the control cohort to evaluate for the presence of any field effect. When a combination of five optical markers was used, all derivatives of 4D-ELF and LEBS, the ability to discern normal control from pancreatic adenocarcinoma occurred with a sensitivity of 95% and specificity of 91%. Discernment between normal and resectable pancreatic adenocarcinoma with this combination of five optical markers resulted in a sensitivity of 100% and specificity of 94%. These five optical markers were spectal slope, fractal dimension, LEBS full width-half max, and LEBS autocorrelation decay (**Fig. 4**). ANOVA and correlation analyses were performed to ensure that the detected differences were not a product of age or smoking history. The diagnostic performance of this test was not altered by tumor size, stage, or location, as, interestingly, even body and tail lesions resulted in the same abnormal fingerprinting despite absence of proximity to the ampulla. Efforts to detect any field effect in the distal duodenum and stomach were negative.[9]

FUTURE DIRECTIONS

Although early approaches to reflectance spectroscopy were based on a simple delivery and collection geometry, new approaches have become more sophisticated and offer the potential for a greater impact. The new advances make use of differential measurements and coherence-based approaches to obtain greater discrimination.

Differential optical pathlength spectroscopy was developed by H.J.C.M. Sternborg from Erasmus University Medical Center, Rotterdam,[10–12] and is an extension of traditional reflectance spectroscopy that uses two closely matched collection paths to

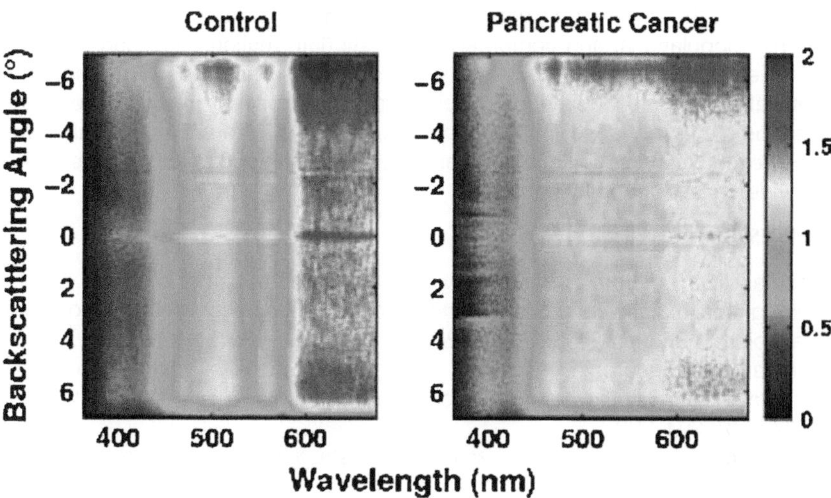

Fig. 4. 4D-ELF detects early increase in blood supply changes even the the duodenal mucosa of pancreatic cancer patients compared to controls.

assess subtle differences in photon migration paths. This approach has been used successfully to detect precancerous lesions in the respiratory tract and could potentially impact GI diagnostics in the future.

Two promising technologies from the group of Vadim Backman at Northwestern University use reflectance spectroscopy for assessing cancer risk. The 4D-ELF technique uses multiple parameters of light scattering to identify diseased tissues. Preliminary results using animal models show that this approach can be used to identify preneoplastic events. Another approach from this group is the LEBS method.[13,14] This technology exploits a coherent effect to isolate light scattering with a specific penetration depth. This approach has been applied to assessing the risk of colon cancer by examining the uninvolved mucosa and presents significant potential as a future screening technique. This diagnostic tool highlights the presence of field "defects" or dysplasia, where, by gross histologic evaluation, tissue is otherwise normal, but interrogation by quantifying red cell count and superficial microvascular patterns reveals preneoplastic changes.

Angle-resolved low coherence interferometry[5,6,15] has been developed by Wax at Duke University as a combination of light scattering and optical coherence tomography. In this modality, depth-resolved nuclear morphology measurements are used to assess tissue health. Greater than 90% sensitivity and specificity for detecting dysplasia have been obtained in ex vivo human tissue studies of Barrett's esophagus tissue.[15] In vivo clinical trials are underway to detect precancerous lesions in Barrett's esophagus patients. Preliminary results that use this approach have been presented at the American Society for Gastrointestinal Endoscopy meeting, indicating high sensitivity and specificity.

SUMMARY

The integration of these technologies into standard endoscopic systems will provide a rapid, accurate, and dependable avenue to evaluate extensive areas of GI tissues. A "heads-up" display on the endoscopic field of view with spectroscopic results of underlying microarchitectural abnormalities will provide for targeting of dysplastic and neoplastic tissue with anticipated greater diagnostic sensitivity, earlier detection in high-risk populations, and computed diagnostic information, removing the risk of sampling error and bringing subjectivity to endoscopic sampling. This model will also obviate the endoscopist from deciphering spectroscopy results. The current point-probe accessory does limit the amount of tissue that can be realistically evaluated; however, when this limitation is overcome, larger fields of tissue will be screened with a wide variety of applications.

REFERENCES

1. Friedland S, Benaron D, Parachikov I, et al. Measurement of mucosal capillary hemoglobin oxygen saturation in the colon by reflectance spectrophotometry. Gastrointest Endosc 2003;57(4):492–7.
2. Friedland S, Benaron D, Coogan S, et al. Diagnosis of chronic mesenteric ischemia by visible light spectroscopy during endoscopy. Gastrointest Endosc 2007;65(2):294–300.
3. Backman V, Wallace MB, Perelman LT, et al. Detection of preinvasive cancer cells. Nature 2000;406(6791):35–6.
4. Wallace MB, Perelman LT, Backman V, et al. Endoscopic detection of dysplasia in patients with Barrett's esophagus using light-scattering spectroscopy. Gastroenterology 2000;119(3):677–82.
5. Wax A, Yang CH, Muller MG, et al. In situ detection of neoplastic transformation and chemopreventive effects in rat esophagus epithelium using angle-resolved low-coherence interferometry. Cancer Res 2003;63(13):3556–9.
6. Wax A, Pyhtila JW, Graf RN, et al. Prospective grading of neoplastic change in rat esophagus epithelium using angle-resolved low-coherence interferometry. J Biomed Opt 2005;10(5):051604.
7. Roy HK, Liu Y, Wali RK, et al. Four-dimensional elastic light-scattering fingerprints as preneoplastic markers in the rat model of colon carcinogenesis. Gastroenterology 2004;126(4):1071–81 [discussion: 948].
8. Wali RK, Roy HK, Kim YL, et al. Increased microvascular blood content is an early event in colon carcinogenesis. Gut 2005;54(5):654–60.
9. Liu Y, Brand RE, Turzhitsky V, et al. Optical markers in duodenal mucosa predict the presence of pancreatic cancer. Clin Cancer Res 2007;13(15 Pt 1):4392–9.
10. Aerts JG, Bard MP, Amelink A, et al. Oxygen saturation measured in vivo in bronchial tumors during bronchoscopy in patients with lung cancer using differential path length spectroscopy (DPS) correlates with survival, stage of the disease, and expression of HIF1a. J Clin Oncol 2006;24(18):5615.
11. Bard MPL, Amelink A, Skurichina M, et al. Optical spectroscopy for the classification of malignant lesions of the bronchial tree. Chest 2006;129(4):995–1001.
12. Amelink A, Sterenborg H, Bard MPL, et al. In vivo measurement of the local optical properties of tissue by use of differential path-length spectroscopy. Opt Lett 2004;29(10):1087–9.
13. Roy HK, Kim YL, Liu Y, et al. Risk stratification of colon carcinogenesis through enhanced backscattering spectroscopy analysis of the uninvolved colonic mucosa. Clin Cancer Res 2006;12(3):961–8.
14. Kim YL, Turzhitsky VM, Liu Y, et al. Low-coherence enhanced backscattering: review of principles and applications for colon cancer screening. J Biomed Opt 2006;11(4):541125.
15. Pyhtila JW, Chalut KJ, Boyer JD, et al. In situ detection of nuclear atypia in Barrett's esophagus using angle-resolved low coherence interferometry. Gastrointest Endosc 2007;65:487–91.

Gastrointestinal Optical Coherence Tomography: Clinical Applications, Limitations, and Research Priorities

Jun Zhang, PhD[a], Zhongping Chen, PhD[a], Gerard Isenberg, MD[b,*]

KEYWORDS

- Optical coherence tomography • Endoscopic imaging
- Imaging technology • Gastrointestinal imaging
- Neoplasia detection

The future ain't what it used to be.
—Yogi Berra

Optical coherence tomography (OCT), a recently developed imaging modality, is based on coherence domain optical technology.[1–4] OCT takes advantage of the short coherence length of broadband light sources to perform micrometer-scale, cross-sectional imaging of biologic tissue. The high spatial resolution of OCT enables noninvasive, in vivo "optical biopsy," and provides immediate and localized diagnostic information. OCT was first used clinically in ophthalmology for the imaging and diagnosis of retinal disease.[2] Recently, it has been applied to imaging of the subsurface structure in skin, vessels, oral cavities, and respiratory, urogenital, and gastrointestinal tracts.[2]

With the resolution one order of magnitude better than that of ultrasound, application of endoscopic OCT in gastrointestinal screening and diagnostics will be a major advance over endoscopic ultrasound. OCT in the gastrointestinal tract can be considered to be in its infancy.[5] Studies with gastrointestinal OCT have focused mostly on

[a] Department of Biomedical Engineering, Beckman Laser Institute, University of California, Irvine, Irvine, CA 92612, USA
[b] Division of Gastroenterology and Hepatology, University Hospitals Case Medical Center, Case Western Reserve University School of Medicine, Wearn 253, 11100 Euclid Avenue, Cleveland, OH 44106, USA
* Corresponding author.
E-mail address: gerard.isenberg@case.edu (G. Isenberg).

Gastrointest Endoscopy Clin N Am 19 (2009) 243–259
doi:10.1016/j.giec.2009.02.003 giendo.theclinics.com
1052-5157/09/$ – see front matter

Barrett's esophagus and the identification of dysplasia.[6–10] There are scattered reports regarding other areas of the gastrointestinal tract, including the colon[11–13] and the pancreaticobiliary duct,[14,15] but these reports represent preliminary work. As technological advancements and experience with this technique progress, the vast potential of OCT is becoming apparent.

Because of issues such as motion artifacts and the need for ease of use, endoscopic OCT imaging of the gastrointestinal tract must be performed in near real time. The effort to attain this goal has been considerable. New technologies using the Fourier domain technique, which measures the magnitude and delay of backscattered light by spectral analysis of the interference pattern, provide 10 to 100 times faster imaging speeds compared with conventional time domain OCT (TDOCT). In addition to advances in optical technology, high-speed electronics and real-time software algorithms for data acquisition, processing, transformation, display, and recording have been developed to realize the goal of real-time endoscopic OCT imaging.

Currently, there are two forms of endoscopic probes, linear scanning and radial scanning. Radial scanning, similar to that used for standard endoscopic ultrasound (EUS) imaging, will prove to be the preferred choice for evaluating the gastrointestinal tract due to its ease of use in orientation to the mucosa and interpretation. The drawback to linear scanning is its small sampling volume, similar to point spectroscopy.

The resolution of OCT is expected to improve with the development of new light sources with broader bandwidth and further advances in software engineering. In a comparative in vivo study, the resolution of a typical current OCT system was about 10 times greater than a 30-MHz ultrasound catheter probe.[16] High-resolution OCT with axial resolution on the order of 1 μm has also been demonstrated by several groups using ultrabroadband light sources.[17] However, few studies have combined high resolution with high speed.

Doppler OCT has also been developed to image vascular structures.[18] Blood flow within vessels and the direction of flow can be measured.[19] Potential applications for Doppler OCT include assessment of bleeding lesions (eg, ulcers, varices, arteriovenous malformations), response to endoscopic treatment,[20] and possibly in the area of tumor angiogenesis.

PRINCIPLES OF OCT

One of the challenges for tomographic imaging of tissue using visible or near-infrared light is tissue optical scattering. When photons propagate inside tissue, they undergo multiple scattering. The mean free path of photons in skin, for example, is 5 μm. If the light is focused 1 mm below the skin surface, most photons undergo multiple scattering and never reach the target point. Less than one in a million photons will reach the target, undergo a single backscattering, and return to the detector. Most photons that are backscattered and reach the detector are multiple scattered photons that do not carry information on the target point. Therefore, the challenge for tomographic imaging of tissues is to separate the single backscattered photons that carry information about the target point from multiple scattered photons that form background noise.

OCT uses coherent gating to discriminate single scattered photons from multiple scattered photons. **Fig. 1** illustrates a TDOCT instrument that uses a fiber optic Michelson interferometer with a broadband light as a source. Light from a broadband, partially coherent source is incident on the beam splitter and split equally between reference and target arms of the interferometer. Light backscattered from the turbid sample recombines with light reflected from the reference arm and forms interference

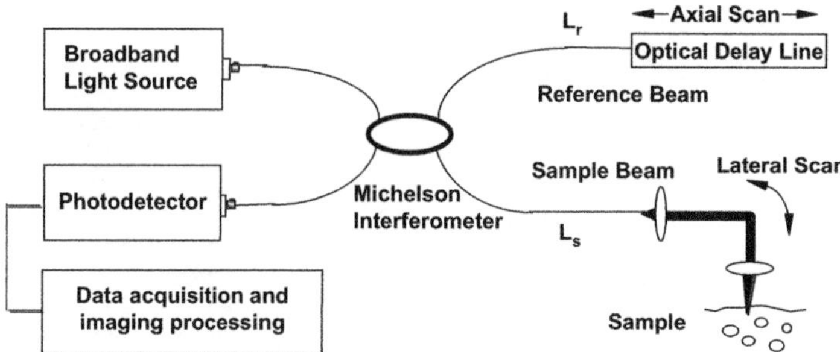

Fig. 1. An OCT system consists of a fiber-based Michelson interferometer with a partially coherent light source.

fringes. High axial spatial resolution is possible because interference fringes are observed only if the path length differences between the sample arm and the reference arm are within the coherence length of the source. The interference fringe intensity signal is amplified, band-pass filtered, and digitized with a high-speed analog-to-digital converter. The signal processing is carried out at the same time as data is transferred to the computer, and real-time display can be accomplished using a digital signal processing board. In the time domain method, axial scans are performed by scanning the reference arm with an optical delay line, and lateral scans are performed by scanning the sample beam. A two-dimensional, cross-sectional image is formed by performing the axial scan followed by a lateral scan. Axial resolution is determined by the coherence length of the source, and lateral resolution is determined by the numerical aperture of the sampling focus lens.

GASTROINTESTINAL TRACT IMAGING WITH OCT

Fig. 2 shows images of the human gastrointestinal tract from endoscopic TDOCT systems[21]. **Fig. 2**A presents OCT images and the corresponding histology of normal colon in vitro. Loss of normal epithelial structure with disruption and disorganization of the crypts is present in images of colon carcinoma (see **Fig. 2**B). **Fig. 2**C shows endoscopic video images of the esophagus and Barrett's esophagus. OCT images of the esophagus and Barrett's esophagus are shown in **Fig. 2**D.

Traditional TDOCT uses a mechanical delay line for depth scanning. Thus, the A-scan rate is limited to less than a few kilohertz. In the Fourier domain method, the reference mirror is fixed, and there is no depth scan. Compared with conventional TDOCT, Fourier domain OCT (FDOCT) measures interference fringes in the spectral domain to reconstruct a tomographic image. Modulation of the interference fringe intensity in the spectral domain is used to determine the locations of all scattering objects along the beam propagation direction by a Fourier transformation. Two methods have been developed to employ the Fourier domain technique: a spectrometer-based system that uses a high-speed line-scan camera[22,23] and a swept laser source-based system that uses a single detector.[24–30] The Fourier domain technique has the advantage of high signal-to-noise ratio compared with the time domain method. In addition, there is no need to scan the reference arm and thus it is capable of unprecedented imaging speed. However, it requires a high-speed spectrometer or a high-speed wavelength swept source.

A schematic diagram of a swept laser source–based Fourier domain OCT system is shown in **Fig. 3**.[29,30] The output light from the swept light source at 1310 nm with a full width half maximum (FWHM) bandwidth of 100 nm and output power of 5 mW is split

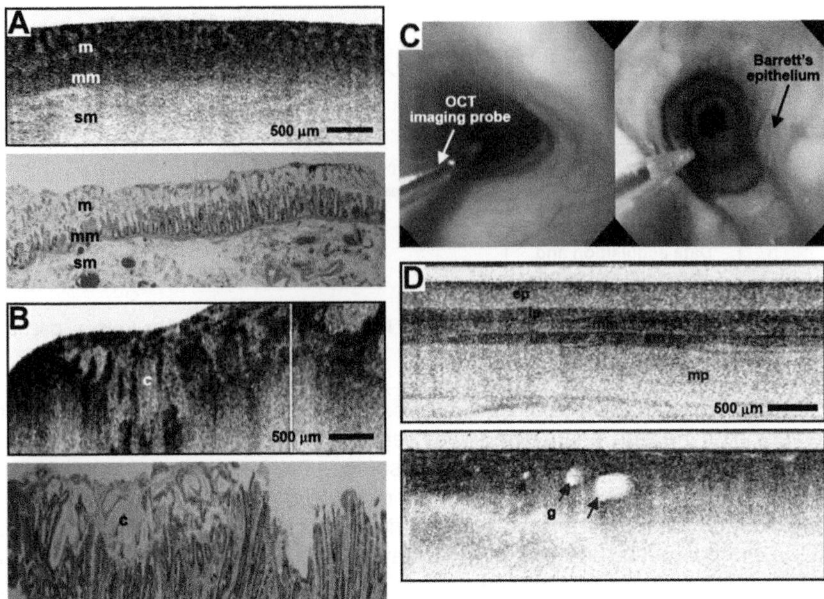

Fig. 2. (*A–D*) OCT imaging of the gastrointestinal tract. (*A, From* Pitris C, Jesser C, Boppart SA, et al. Feasibility of optical coherence tomography for high-resolution imaging of human gastrointestinal tract malignancies. J Gastroenterol 2000;35:87–92; with permission; *B, From* Fujimoto J. Optical coherence tomography for ultrahigh resolution in vivo imaging. Nat Biotechnol 2003;21:1361–7; with permission; *C, From* Li XD, Boppart SA, Van Dam J, et al. Optical coherence tomography: advanced technology for the endoscopic imaging of Barrett's esophagus. Endoscopy. 2000;32:921–30; with permission.)

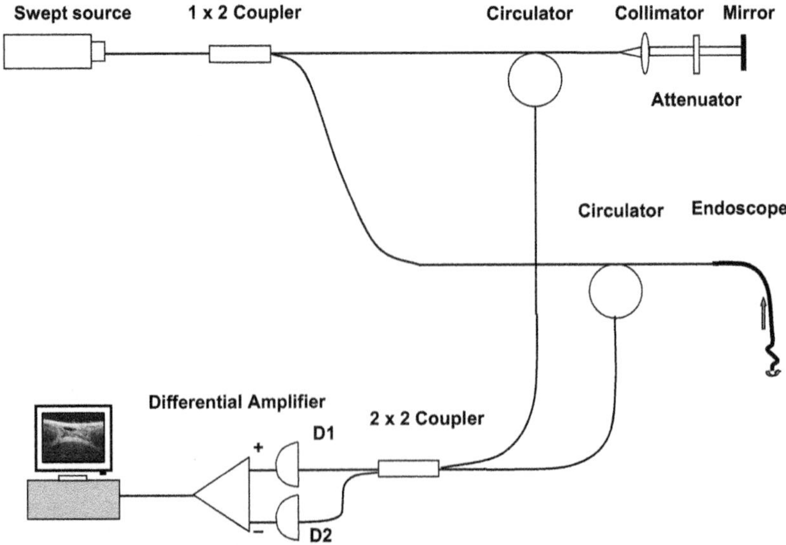

Fig. 3. A fiber-based swept source OCT system.

into reference and sample arms by a 1 × 2 coupler. The light source is operated at a sweeping rate of 20,000 Hz. Eighty percent of the incident power is coupled into the sample arm and 20% is fed into the reference arm. The reference power is attenuated by an adjustable neutral density attenuator for maximum sensitivity. Two circulators are used in the reference and sample arms to redirect the back-reflected light to a 2 × 2 fiber coupler (50:50 split ratio) for balanced detection. To cancel the distortion originating from the nonlinearities in the wave number function $k(t)$, the data are numerically remapped from uniform time to uniform wave number space, based on the function of $k(t)$, which is determined by the spectra calibration process provided by calibration comb signals generated from a fiber Fabry-Perot interferometer. Dispersion calibration is also performed at this step by adding a wave number-dependent phase term. The fast Fourier transform (FFT) performed in k space retrieves the complex depth-encoded fringe signal $\tilde{S}(z)=A(z)\ e^{i\phi(z)}$, which contains the amplitude term $A(z)$ and phase term $\phi(z)$. The structure image can be acquired from the amplitude term. The axial resolution of the system was measured to be 8.5 μm.

A microelectromechanical system (MEMS), rotational, motor-based endoscope is connected to the sample arm. To image the gastrointestinal tract, for example, the esophagus, a rotational scan mode OCT endoscope is more suitable than a linear scanning probe. In conventional OCT endoscope designs using a fixed gradient-index (GRIN) lens and prism as the optics tip, rotational torque is transferred from the endoscope's proximal end to the distal tip. The new rotational MEMS motor-based endoscope design eliminates the rotation of the whole endoscope by rotating only the optical tip of the endoscope. Thus, the related polarization effect of the spinning image probe is eliminated. With the advantage of MEMS technology, the endoscope has a small diameter, which is suitable for many clinical applications. Furthermore, this design can be used with more flexible materials without the need for rotational torque transfer.

The MEMS motor-based OCT endoscope is shown in **Fig. 4**.[29,30] The distal end is enclosed by round-shaped, medical, ultraviolet glue to reduce tissue damage when the probe is advanced into the internal organ. Inside the biocompatible fluorinated ethylene-propylene (FEP) tube, a tiny MEMS motor is backward mounted at the distal end of the probe and is driven by the outside motor controller through a control wire. The 1310-nm single mode fiber is cut to 8° and glued to a focusing GRIN lens. The focused beam is reflected by a right-angle microprism, which is glued to the motor shaft toward the sample. The motor rotation in the current design is much more stable through the cycle feedback control, which is critical for synchronization in three-dimensional slice image acquisition. In addition, the MEMS motor is more robust with an outside steel sheath, which strengthens the connection between the gear head and rotational shaft. The endoscope is fixed to a linear transverse scan stage

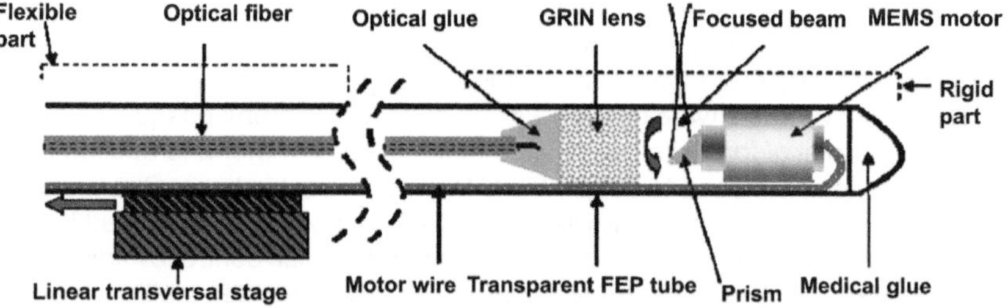

Fig. 4. A three-dimensional MEMS motor-based endoscope. (*From* Su J, Zhang J, Yu L, et al. In vivo three-dimensional microelectromechanical endoscopic swept source optical coherence tomography. Opt Express 2007;15:10390–6; with permission.)

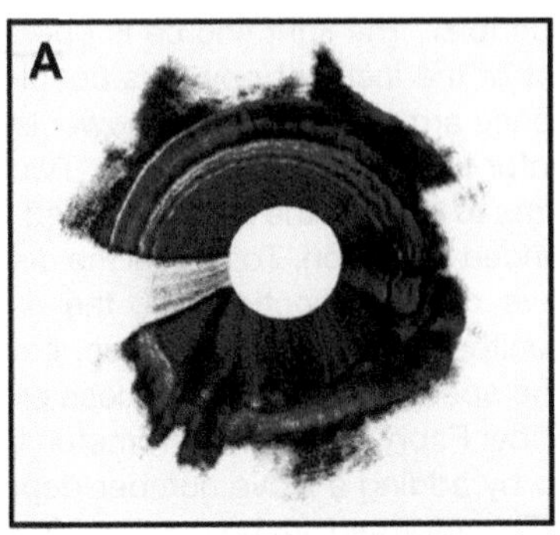

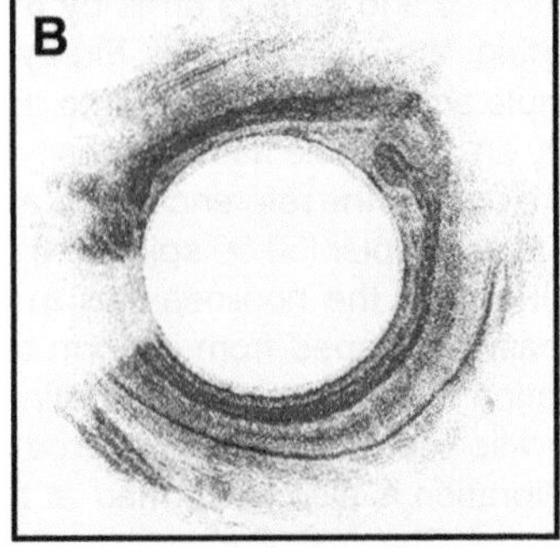

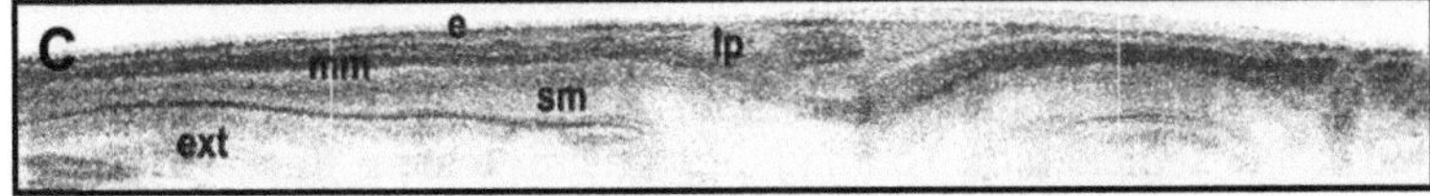

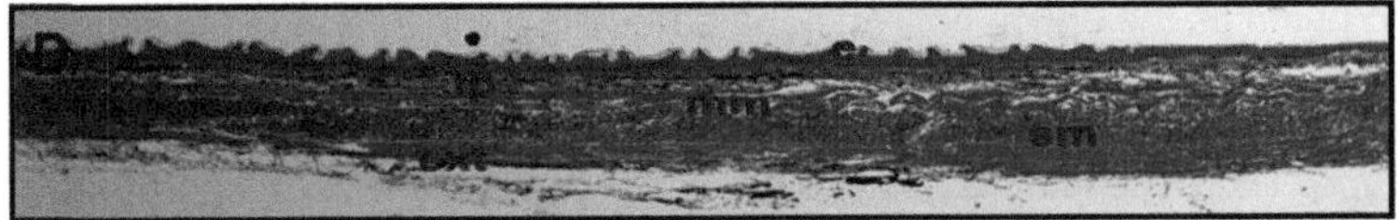

Fig. 5. In vivo OCT study of the rabbit esophagus. (*A*) Three-dimensional rebuilt image of rabbit esophagus, 6-mm long. (*B*) One cross-sectional slice taken from (*A*). (*C*) The transverse image unwrapped from (*B*), size is 9.86 mm by 1.85 mm. (*D*) The histology image at position corresponding to (*C*). (e, epithelium; lp, lamina propria; mm, muscularis mucosae; sm, submucosa; ext, muscularis propria). (*From* Su J, Zhang J, Yu L, et al. In vivo three-dimensional microelectromechanical endoscopic swept source optical coherence tomography. Opt Express 2007; 15:10390–6; with permission.)

at the proper point. To create a three-dimensional helix scan, the whole probe is pulled back slowly by a linear scan stage and the prism is rotated rapidly by the MEMS motor.

In vivo, rabbit GI tracts were imaged in three-dimensional mode with an endoscopic probe based on a 2.2-mm micromotor.[29] **Fig. 5**A shows a three-dimensional volume image of a rabbit esophagus in vivo. **Fig. 5**B shows one of the cross-sectional images sliced from the three-dimensional volume. The 9.86-mm by 1.85-mm transverse slice from **Fig. 5**B is shown unwrapped in **Fig. 5**C. The histologic result at the corresponding location of **Fig. 5**C is shown in **Fig. 5**D. From the unwrapped transverse slice, the layer epithelium, lamina propria, muscularis mucosae, submucosa and muscularis propria are obvious and match well with the histologic result.

Rabbit colon was also imaged with the endoscopic OCT system as shown in **Fig. 6**.

In vivo human GI tracts were imaged with an endoscopic probe based on a 1.5-mm micromotor. A total of four wires were used to connect the motor and outside control circuit. Two wires were used to supply the 3-V direct current voltage. One wire transferred the revolutions per minute (RPM) signal back and one wire controlled the rotational direction. The outside circuit implemented the feedback control by adjusting the supply voltage according to the RPM signal, which increased the stability of the rotational speed. A 2-stage, 40:1 ratio micro-gear head was put in front of the rotational shaft to smooth the step motion, which was designed to achieve an optimal rotational speed at 30 frames per second. In the experiment, the motor speed was set to 19.5

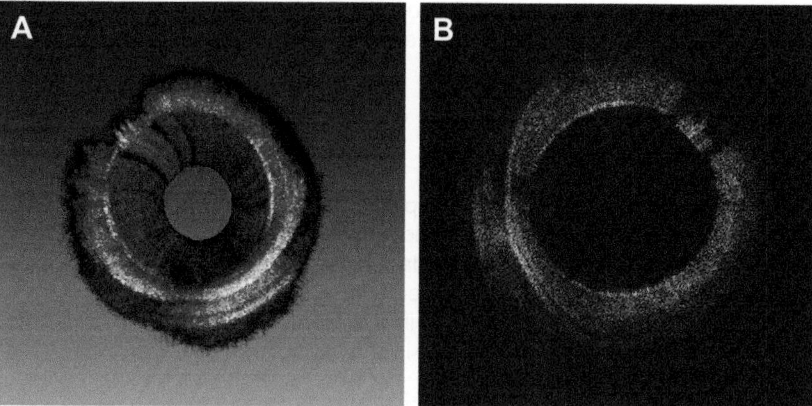

Fig. 6. In vivo OCT study of the rabbit colon. (*A*) Three-dimensional volume image of the rabbit colon. (*B*) One cross-sectional slice taken from (*A*).

frames per second to synchronize with the speed of the OCT system. The outside linear transverse stage pulled the whole endoscope back at 0.4 mm per second to realize a three-dimensional helix scan. A total of 400 image slices were processed and displayed in 20.5 seconds.[30] In the detection arm, the signal collected by the photodetectors was digitized by a 14-bit data acquisition board sampling at 25 million samples per second, and the number of data points for each axial line (A-line) data acquisition was 1024. The A-line data acquisition start trigger for the digitizer was generated by the swept source. The digitizer outputted the A-line data directly to a digital signal processor (DSP) board through a custom-designed auxiliary bus. The complex, analytical, depth-encoded signal was converted from the collected detection signal by calibration, dispersion compensation, and FFT. The structure image was reconstructed from the amplitude term of the complex depth-encoded signal. In the DSP board, eight DSPs were programmed to work in parallel to implement the algorithm. The digitized data were fed sequentially into the DSP board from the digitizer. Each DSP handled a 1024 A-line image frame independently, with the help of a scheduler. The resulting structural image was sent to the monitor, in the same order as the input. The processing power from the DSPs handled a 20-kHz A-line easily.[30] **Fig. 7** shows in vivo endoscopic FDOCT imaging of a human

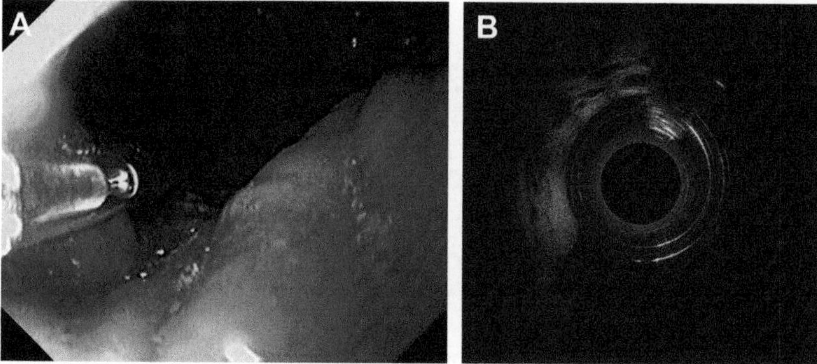

Fig. 7. In vivo OCT study of the human stomach. (*A*) OCT MEMS probe on top of a polyp. (*B*) Polyp OCT image.

stomach with a polyp structure. **Fig. 8** shows in vivo endoscopic FDOCT imaging of human esophagus. Layers of epithelium are present in an OCT image of a normal esophagus (see **Fig. 8**A).

CLINICAL APPLICATIONS

Potentially, OCT has an important role in the management of patients with gastro-intestinal disorders characterized by dysplasia, particularly those in which there is a continuum from dysplasia to cancer, and especially if these lesions are small, and difficult or impossible to detect with standard endoscopic imaging techniques.

OCT may not replace biopsy and histopathologic evaluation, but it will likely bring endoscopy and histopathology together in a single technology. Clearly, the future OCT endoscopist will need to be trained in the histopathologic changes that occur in tissue damage or dysplasia.

As shown in preliminary studies,[10] OCT could play a significant role in targeting specific sites for mucosal biopsies. In theory, OCT could actually eliminate the need for biopsies in the surveillance of precancerous conditions, such as Barrett's esophagus or chronic ulcerative colitis, or at least reduce the number of biopsies required in standard protocols. There is also the potential for OCT to guide therapy for these conditions.

Barrett's Esophagus

Barrett's esophagus is readily identified by OCT.[5–9] Usually, Barrett's esophagus is easily suspected endoscopically with the presence of pink salmon-colored mucosa above the end of the gastric folds within the esophagus. However, in some cases of short-segment Barrett's esophagus, the squamocolumnar junction may not be obvious endoscopically, and OCT may be valuable in identifying intestinal metaplasia in these cases.

Dysplasia in Barrett's esophagus is histopathologically identified by characteristic cytologic and architectural changes. A study evaluating the accuracy of OCT in the diagnosis of dysplasia in Barrett's esophagus revealed an accuracy rate of 70% as interpreted by the endoscopists.[10] However, there was a high negative predictive value (91%) suggesting that OCT could be used to target biopsies in areas of Barrett's esophagus with a higher probability for the presence of dysplasia. Certainly, as

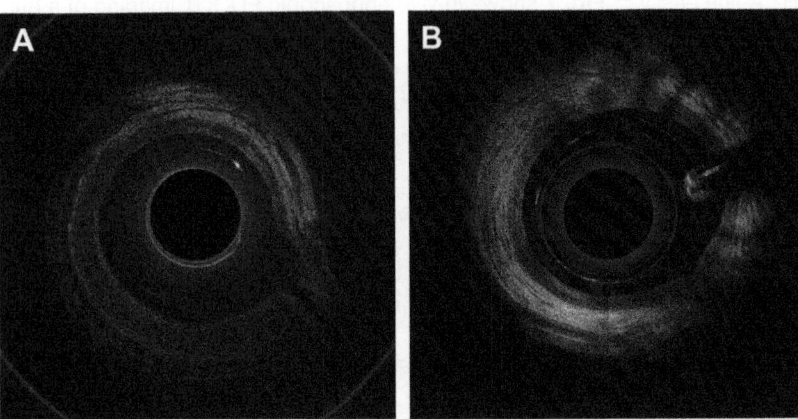

Fig. 8. In vivo OCT study of the human esophagus. (*A*) OCT image. (*B*) OCT image at another site.

endoscopists' experience with performing OCT and their interpretative skills improve, it can be expected that accuracy rates will improve. Currently, two features seem to be specific for dysplasia and cancer in OCT imaging: (1) focal (dark) areas of decreased light scattering; (2) focal loss of mucosal structure and organization.[6] **Fig. 9** depicts OCT images of normal esophagus and Barrett's esophagus with various degrees of dysplasia.

Clarification regarding which particular OCT characteristics for dysplasia in Barrett's esophagus are more important and whether there are other heretofore unrecognized features that imply dysplasia may improve overall sensitivity, specificity, and accuracy. Computer digital analysis with a neural network was used to evaluate the same OCT images obtained in Isenberg's study.[10] The computer's accuracy rate was found to be 94%, suggesting that computers may enhance image evaluation to the extent that the endoscopist is not needed for interpretation.[31] It is likely that using computer protocols on a real-time basis for interpretation will allow OCT to be used quickly and efficiently to survey patients with Barrett's esophagus. With innovations in the endoscopic OCT probe that will allow complete imaging of the esophagus despite peristalsis or respiratory movements in combination with computer-driven protocols for interpretation, it may be possible to survey the esophagus for dysplasia in 1 to 2 minutes. A pilot study with high-speed OCT technology using optical

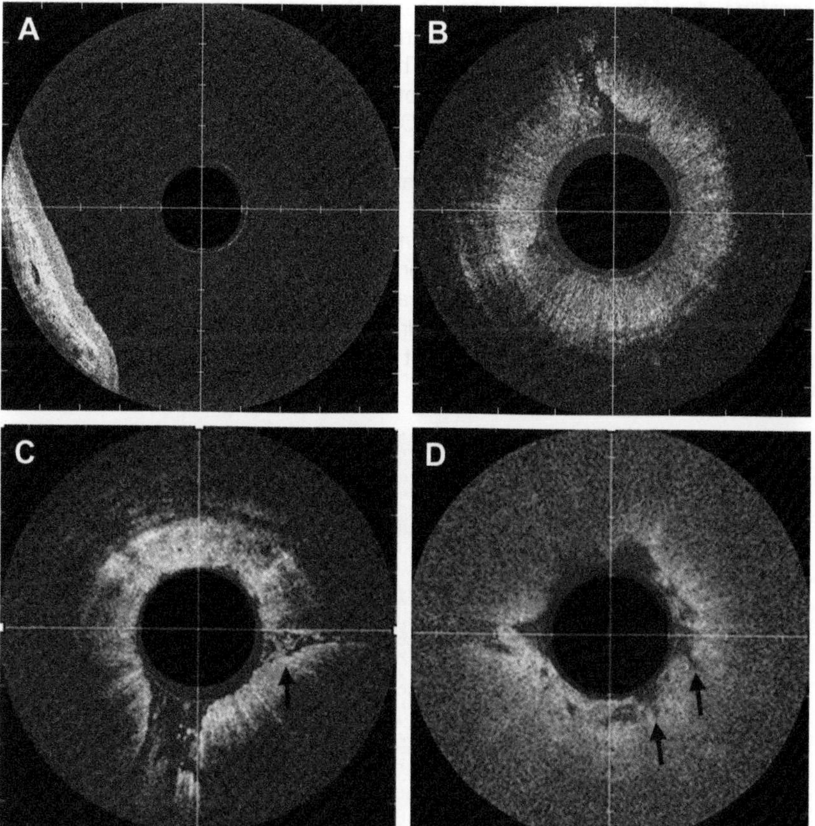

Fig. 9. OCT images of normal esophagus (*A*) and Barrett's esophagus with low-grade dysplasia (*B*), high-grade dysplasia (*C*), and intramucosal cancer (*D*).

frequency domain imaging and a balloon-centering catheter in 10 patients demonstrated the feasibility of obtaining OCT images of an approximately 6-cm length of distal esophagus within 2 minutes.[32]

OCT may also be useful in identifying structural changes after ablative therapy for Barrett's esophagus. Endoscopic ablation is performed to induce a reversion of specialized intestinal metaplasia to squamous or neosquamous epithelium. This reversion is believed to reduce the risk of adenocarcinoma. Although ablative therapy in its various forms can induce a neosquamous mucosa, whether and to what extent the risk for cancer is reduced is uncertain. It is clear, however, that cancer can arise beneath the neosquamous epithelium. OCT might be used to assess the results of ablative therapy and detect insufficiently treated areas.[9] Similarly, OCT could be used to identify the resection margins of lesions treated with endoscopic mucosectomy to ensure that they are clear.

Stomach

For reasons yet to be determined, the best quality OCT images obtained in the gastrointestinal tract are from the esophagus and the colon. Images from the stomach are less satisfactory as the depth of penetration is reduced, which may be secondary to the mucus layer. **Fig. 10** depicts OCT images of the stomach. Further work is needed to clarify why OCT imaging is not as ideal in the stomach.

Propylene glycol has been used as a contrast agent in conjunction with OCT and provides a more detailed visualization of the microstructures in resected specimens of human esophagus and stomach.[33] The physical basis for this enhancement remains to be determined. Presumably, other agents or dyes might be found that would be better suited to the purpose of OCT image enhancement. It remains to be seen whether this agent would be effective and safe in vivo. Certainly, the use of contrasting agents in the stomach and other areas of the gastrointestinal tract warrants further investigation.

OCT could possibly identify premalignant lesions or conditions potentially predisposing to malignancy, such as gastric intestinal metaplasia, gastritis associated with *Helicobacter pylori*, and early gastric cancer involving the mucosa or submucosa. In addition, OCT may be useful for detecting residual tumor in lesions removed with endoscopic mucosectomy, similar to that of the esophagus or other areas of the gastrointestinal tract.

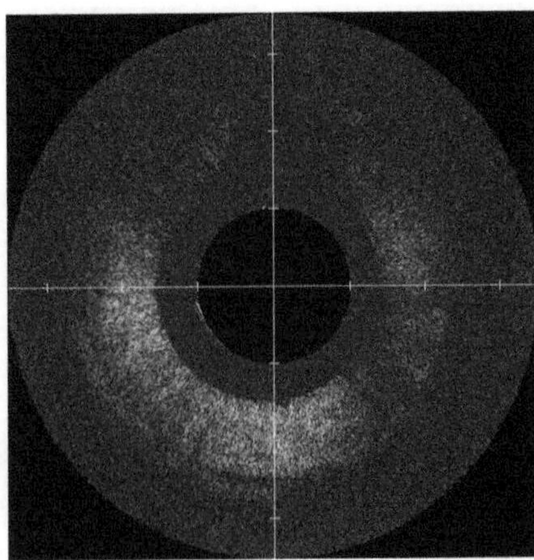

Fig. 10. OCT image of a normal stomach.

Small Intestine

The villous structure of the small intestine is easily seen with OCT,[12] implying that OCT may potentially identify patients with celiac sprue. In addition, dysplastic features at the ampulla may be identified in patients at risk (eg, patients with familial adenomatous polyposis), which would allow for earlier intervention.

Colon

There is vast potential for OCT imaging of the colon, including the possibility of differentiating between ulcerative colitis and Crohn's disease in patients presenting with inflammatory bowel disease, identifying dysplasia in surveillance programs for these patients, and determining whether a particular polyp needs to be removed. OCT can differentiate adenomatous polyps from hyperplastic polyps (**Fig. 11**).[11]

Practical benefits include avoiding the risk of unnecessary polypectomy, thereby saving time and cost associated with the histopathologic assessment currently needed for all colon polyps. In addition, the risk of bleeding, infection, and perforation associated with the unnecessary polypectomy would be eliminated. OCT could potentially identify smaller, flat adenomas that may be missed at standard endoscopy. OCT may be a more effective and efficient substitute for high-magnification endoscopy and chromoendoscopy. In addition, the detection of aberrant crypt foci, which are considered dysplastic, may allow risk stratification of patients who would benefit from screening or surveillance colonoscopy.

Pancreaticobiliary

Most pancreatic cancers arise from ductal epithelium in which dysplastic changes have been identified histologically as the microscopic precursors of invasive adenocarcinoma. Similarly, because of ongoing chronic inflammation and reparative changes that occur in primary sclerosing cholangitis (PSC), the biliary epithelium undergoes progressive dysplastic changes and cholangiocarcinoma frequently results. Available imaging techniques (eg, intraductal ultrasound, endoscopic retrograde cholangiopancreatography [ERCP], magnetic resonance cholangiopancreatography [MRCP]) are inadequate for identifying these dysplastic lesions before cancer develops. Thus, improved techniques for ductal imaging, such as OCT, at a resolution that defines cellular structure would be of substantial benefit. Other areas of interest

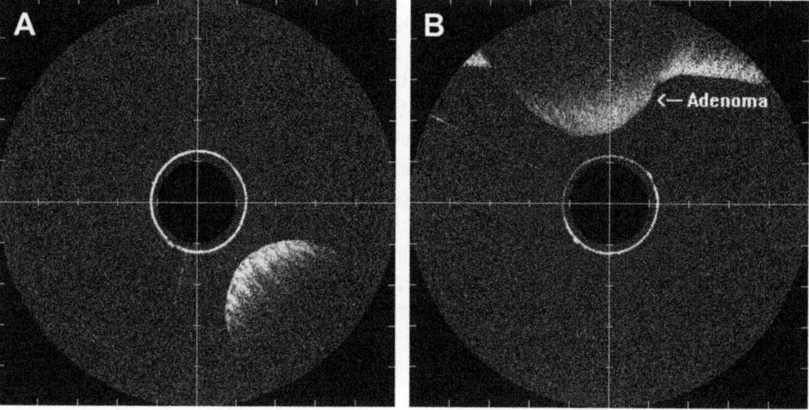

Fig. 11. OCT images of a hyperplastic polyp (*A*) and an adenomatous polyp (*B*).

include differentiating benign strictures in terms of prognostic potential for endoscopic versus surgical therapy, such as those that can occur in liver transplant patients, and evaluating the pancreatic duct epithelium in patients with chronic pancreatitis to determine correlation with secretory function. **Fig. 12** shows OCT images of normal epithelium and various degrees of dysplasia, including pancreatic, intraductal, papillary mucinous neoplasia and malignancy.

The proper role of OCT in the diagnostic algorithm vis-à-vis EUS, ERCP, and cholangiopancreatoscopy will need to be established. Technologic considerations of OCT imaging within the bile duct and pancreatic duct will need to be evaluated, including the proper focal length and optimal wavelength needed for accurate imaging. In a pilot study, OCT was superior to brush cytology in distinguishing nonneoplastic from neoplastic main pancreatic duct strictures.[34] Another study showed that intraductal OCT accurately identified dysplastic changes or cancer in the bile duct and pancreatic duct during ERCP in 22 patients.[35]

COMBINING HIGH RESOLUTION WITH HIGH SPEED FOR ENDOSCOPIC GASTROINTESTINAL OCT

Clinical applications of endoscopic gastrointestinal OCT require high speed and high resolution. Enhancing the resolution of OCT is important for early diagnosis of disease, such as cancer. With the enhanced axial resolution of 3 μm and below, it is possible to obtain in vivo OCT tomograms close to the level of histology.[17] Such a high spatial resolution would greatly increase the capability of OCT for early detection of cancer. However, high-resolution OCT imaging is difficult to perform with high speed.

The axial resolution of a swept source-based FDOCT system is determined by the sweeping bandwidth of the source. Thus, a broadband swept source is required to build a high-resolution FDOCT system. Currently, several commercial swept light sources have been reported. These swept laser sources incorporate a semiconductor optical amplifier (SOA) gain medium with a tunable optical band-pass filter in the cavity, which has the drawbacks of a limited FWHM sweeping bandwidth (<100 nm) due to the narrow bandwidth of a conventional SOA (~75 nm) and a limited tuning rate (<28 kHz) due to the long characteristic time constant for building up laser activity inside the cavity.

The limited tuning rate can be overcome with the new Fourier domain mode locking (FDML) technique by extending the laser cavity and periodically driving the optical band-pass filter synchronously with the optical round-trip time of the propagating light wave in the cavity.[28] This permits broad sweep ranges, narrow instantaneous linewidths, and unprecedented sweep rates. In addition, the phase stability of the system can be significantly increased because the FDML swept source operates in a quasi-stationary regime.

A broadband FDML swept source operated at a turning speed of 47 kHz has been developed combining two SOAs as the gain medium.[36] This broadband FDML laser permits high-resolution imaging with high speed. The swept laser source with parallel configuration of two SOAs is shown in **Fig. 13**. The FDML wavelength swept laser consists of two SOAs, two isolators, two 3-dB fiber couplers, two polarization controllers, a scanning fiber Fabry-Perot tunable filter (FFP-TF), and a 4.5-km-long SMF-28e dispersion managed fiber. In this experiment, the parallel scheme is adopted because the serial configuration has a problem in that each SOA exhibits absorption in the portion of the spectrum outside of its unique gain band.[37] The center wavelengths of the SOAs are 1272 nm and 1322 nm. The FFP-TF has a free spectral range of approximately 210 nm at 1300 nm and a linewidth of approximately 0.2 nm. The applied frequency of the FFP-TF is 45.6 kHz, which is the same as the fundamental

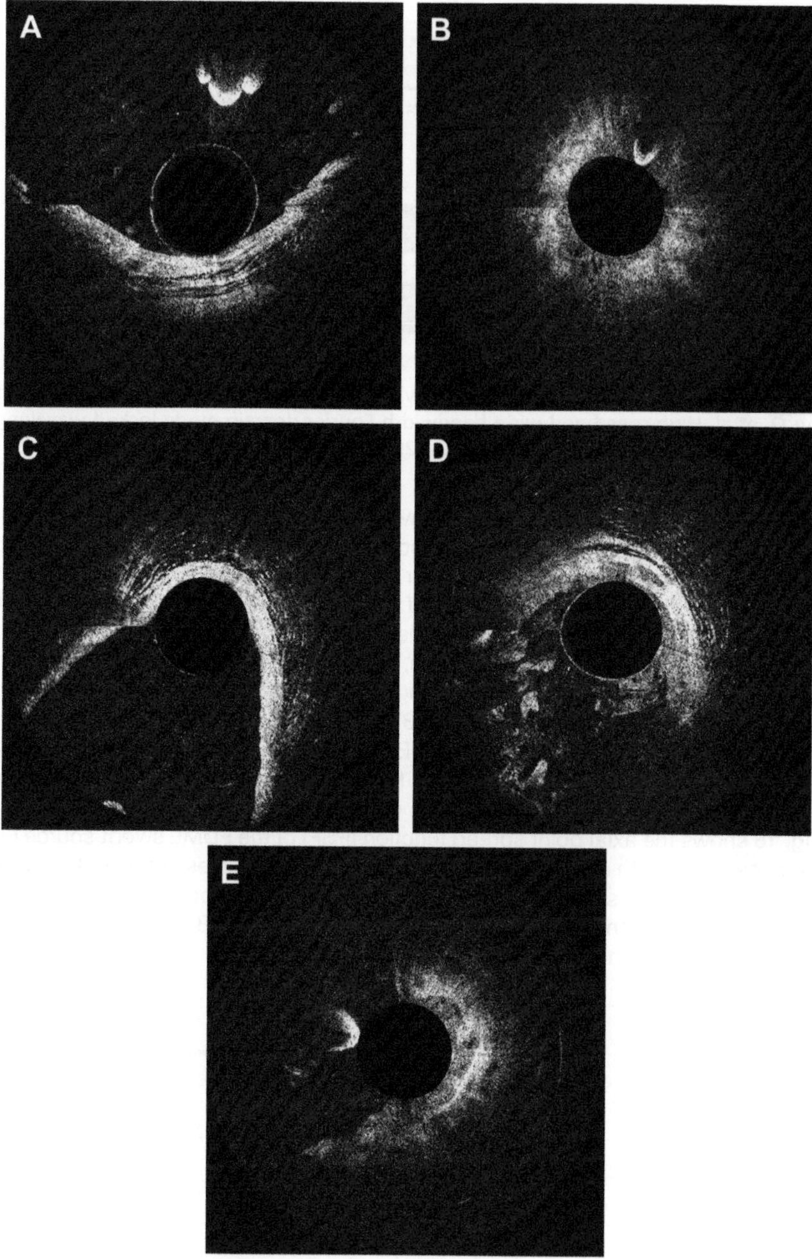

Fig. 12. Intraductal OCT images of normal bile duct epithelium (*A*), cholangiocarcinoma (*B*), normal pancreatic duct (*C*), pancreatic intraductal papillary mucinous neoplasia (*D*), and pancreatic adenocarcinoma (*E*).

longitudinal frequency of the total laser cavity. Polarization controllers are inserted into the laser cavity because both SOAs are polarization dependent. The pigtailed fiber length of each SOA should be the same in order to match the longitudinal frequency of each laser cavity. Two isolators are used to operate unidirectional propagation in

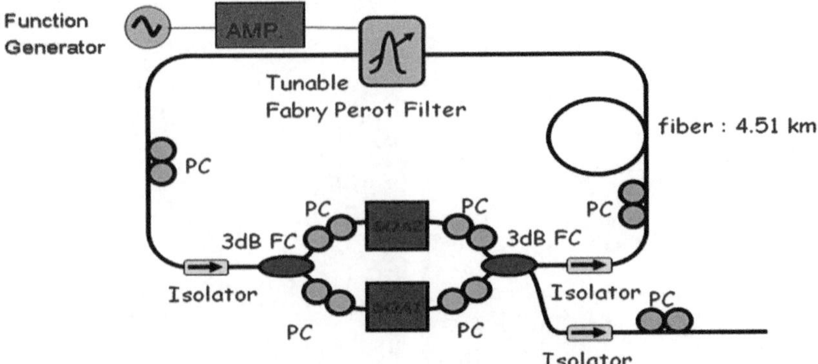

Fig. 13. The broadband FDML swept source with multiple SOAs. (*From* Jeon MY, Zhang J, Wang Q, et al. High-speed and wide bandwidth Fourier domain mode-locked wavelength swept laser with multiple SOAs. Opt Express 2008;16:2547–54; with permission.)

the laser cavities. The output from the wavelength swept laser is monitored with an optical spectrum analyzer and an oscilloscope using a 3-dB fiber coupler. The output of the FDML laser is coupled into a Fourier domain OCT imaging system.

Fig. 14 shows the laser output spectra of the FDML wavelength swept sources with different SOAs. The 3-dB tuning range of the swept source with only the shorter wavelength SOA is 72 nm from 1241 to 1313 nm. The edge-to-edge tuning range is 108 nm from 1220 to 1328 nm. The 3-dB tuning range of the swept source with only the longer wavelength SOA is 63 nm from 1314 to 1377 nm. The edge-to-edge tuning range is 102 nm from 1278 to 1380 nm. The 3 dB tuning range of the swept source with combined SOAs is 132 nm from 1245 to 1377 nm. The edge-to-edge tuning range is 160 nm from 1220 to 1380 nm.

Fig. 15 shows the axial point spread function (PSF) of the FDML swept source OCT system measured with a partial reflector. The measured axial resolution of the system is 6.6 μm in air corresponding to an effective axial resolution of 4.7 μm in tissue (n = 1.4). The instantaneous linewidth is determined to be 0.18 nm by measuring the coherence length of the laser.

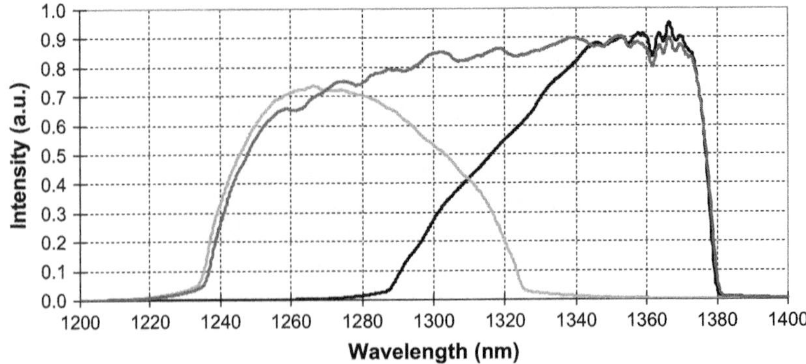

Fig. 14. Optical spectra of FDML swept sources. Light gray line, optical spectrum of the swept source with only the shorter wavelength SOA; black line, optical spectrum of the swept source with only the longer wavelength SOA; dark gray line, optical spectrum of the swept source with combined SOAs.

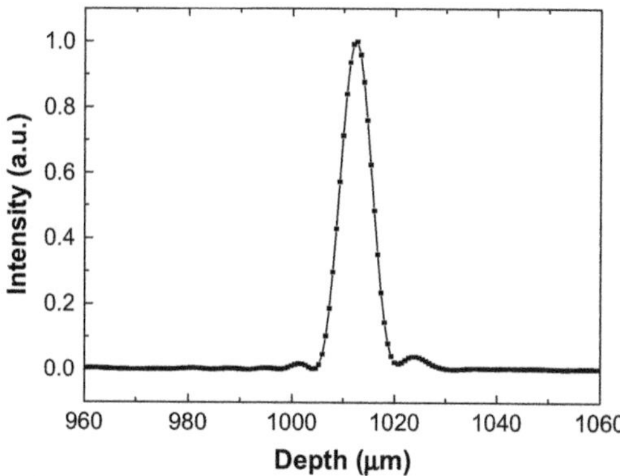

Fig. 15. Forward scan PSF of the FDML swept source OCT system. (*From* Jeon MY, Zhang J, Wang Q, et al. High-speed and wide bandwidth Fourier domain mode-locked wavelength swept laser with multiple SOAs. Opt Express 2008;16:2547–54; with permission.)

A swept source with broader bandwidth can be achieved by combining three or more parallel SOAs with different center wavelengths as the gain medium. Hence an ultrahigh speed, high-resolution, three-dimensional endoscopic FDOCT system can be built based on the fast scanning, broad bandwidth, FDML swept source.

SUMMARY

OCT provides the highest resolution available of any of the technologies currently used in endoscopic imaging. There are several potential clinical applications for OCT, particularly with precancerous conditions of the gastrointestinal tract. Priorities for research include technologic improvements in improving resolution to the cellular and subcellular levels while maintaining high imaging speed. Doppler and spectroscopic OCT need to be further evaluated as these applications may provide functional imaging. Development of swept sources with broad scanning range and rapid scanning rate is critical for high speed, high-resolution OCT imaging. Rapid image acquisition through improvements in probe design and software programming is necessary to reduce procedural time. Safety in terms of light exposure to the gastrointestinal mucosa needs to be elucidated and standardized. Dysplasia needs to better clarified in terms of OCT features. Computer-aided diagnosis may eliminate the need for intensive training of endoscopists on interpretation and allow ease of use.

Currently, a few preliminary clinical studies involving small numbers of patients have been published. Larger, carefully conducted, prospective trials are needed to determine the clinical usefulness of this imaging modality. In particular, clinical research priorities should focus on Barrett's esophagus, colon polyps, aberrant crypt foci, inflammatory bowel disease, and pancreaticobiliary neoplasia. The clinical usefulness of contrast agents, including the use of nanoshells (nanotechnology) and protein-coated microspheres, needs to be evaluated. Comparison of OCT either in combination or in contrast with other imaging technologies such as fluorescence and confocal microscopy is needed. Finally, cost-effectiveness needs to be established. OCT may become either a primary or adjunctive tool for endoscopic imaging, depending on the indication. As advances in technology occur and techniques become more refined, the future of OCT, in the vein of Yogi Berra's philosophy, will likely change.

REFERENCES

1. Huang D, Swanson EA, Lin CP, et al. Optical coherence tomography. Science 1991;254(5035):1178–81.
2. Bouma BE, Tearney GJ. Handbook of optical coherence tomography. New York: Marcel Dekker; 2002.
3. Fercher AF, Hitzenberger CK. Optical coherence tomography. In: Wolf E, editor. Progress in optics, vol. 44. Amsterdam: Elsevier; 2002. p. 215–302.
4. Chen Z. Functional optical coherence tomgoraphy. In: Hwang NHC, Woo SL-Y, editors. Frontiers in biomedical engineering. New York: Kluwer Academic/Plenum; 2003. p. 345–64.
5. Isenberg G, Sivak MJ. Gastrointestinal optical coherence tomography. Tech Gastrointest Endosc 2003;2:94–101.
6. Das A, Sivak MV Jr, Chak A, et al. Role of high-resolution endoscopic imaging using optical coherence tomography in patients with Barrett's esophagus. Gastrointest Endosc 2000;51:AB93.
7. Poneros JM, Brand S, Bouma SE, et al. Diagnosis of specialized intestinal metaplasia by optical coherence tomography. Gastroenterology 2001;120(1):7–12.
8. Jackle S, Gladkova N, Feldchtein F, et al. In vivo endoscopic optical coherence tomography of esophagitis, Barrett's esophagus, and adenocarcinoma of the esophagus. Endoscopy 2000;32:750–5.
9. Li XD, Boppart SA, Van Dam J, et al. Optical coherence tomography: advanced technology for the endoscopic imaging of Barrett's esophagus. Endoscopy 2000;32:921–30.
10. Isenberg G, Sivak MV Jr, Chak A, et al. Accuracy of endoscopic optical coherence tomography in the detection of dysplasia in Barrett's esophagus a prospective, double-blinded study. Gastrointest Endosc 2005;62:825–31.
11. Pfau P, Sivak MV Jr, Chak A, et al. Criteria for the diagnosis of dysplasia by endoscopic optical coherence tomography. Gastrointest Endosc 2003;58:196–202.
12. Sivak MV Jr, Kobayashi MV, Izatt JA, et al. High-resolution endoscopic imaging of the GI tract using optical coherence tomography. Gastrointest Endosc 2000;51(4 Pt 1):474–9.
13. Kobayashi K, Izatt JA, Kulkarni MD, et al. High-resolution cross-sectional imaging of the gastrointestinal tract using optical coherence tomography: preliminary results. Gastrointest Endosc 1998;47:515–23.
14. Poneros J, Tearney GJ, Shiskov M, et al. Optical coherence tomography of the biliary tree during ERCP. Gastrointest Endosc 2002;55:84–8.
15. Seitz U, Freund J, Jaeckle S, et al. First in vivo optical coherence tomography in the human bile duct. Endoscopy 2001;33:1018–21.
16. Das A, Sivak MV Jr, Chak A, et al. High resolution endoscopic imaging of the gastrointestinal tract: a comparative study of optical coherence tomography versus high-frequency catheter probe endoscopic ultrasonography. Gastrointest Endosc 2001;54:219–24.
17. Drexler W. Ultrahigh-resolution optical coherence tomography. J Biomed Opt 2004;9:47–74.
18. Chen Z, Milner TE, Wang X, et al. Optical Doppler tomography: imaging in vivo blood flow dynamics following pharmacological intervention and photodynamic therapy. Photochem Photobiol 1998;67:56–60.
19. Ren H, Breke MK, Ding Z, et al. Imaging and quantifying transverse flow velocity with the Doppler bandwidth in a phase-resolved functional optical coherence tomography. Opt Lett 2002;27:409–11.

20. Wong R, Yazdanfar S, Izatt JA, et al. Visualization of subsurface blood vessels by color Doppler optical coherence tomography in rats: before and after hemostatic therapy. Gastrointest Endosc 2002;55:88–95.
21. Fujimoto J. Optical coherence tomography for ultrahigh resolution in vivo imaging. Nat Biotechnol 2003;21:1361–7.
22. Wojtkowski M, Srinivasan VJ, Ko T, et al. Ultrahigh-resolution high speed Fourier domain optical coherence tomography and methods for dispersion compensation. Opt Express 2004;12:2404–22.
23. Cense B, Nassif N, Chen TC, et al. Ultrahigh-resolution high-speed retinal imaging using spectral-domain optical coherence tomgoraphy. Opt Lett 2004; 12:2435–47.
24. Yun SH, Tearney GJ, de Boer JF, et al. High speed optical frequency domain imaging. Opt Express 2003;11:2953–63.
25. Yun SH, Boudoux C, Tearney GJ, et al. High-speed wavelength-swept semiconductor laser with a polygon-scanner-based wavelength filter. Opt Lett 2003;28: 1981–3.
26. Zhang J, Nelson JS, Chen Z. Removal of mirror image and enhancement of signal to noise ratio in Fourier domain optical coherence tomography using an electro-optical phase modulator. Opt Lett 2005;30:147–9.
27. Zhang J, Nelson JS, Chen Z. Full range polarization-sensitive Fourier domain optical coherence tomography. Opt Express 2004;12:6033–9.
28. Huber R, Wojtkowski M, Fujimoto JG. Fourier domain mode locking (FDML): a new laser operating regime and applications for optical coherence tomography. Opt Express 2006;14:3225–37.
29. Su J, Zhang J, Yu L, et al. In vivo three-dimensional microelectromechanical endoscopic swept source optical coherence tomography. Opt Express 2007; 15:10390–6.
30. Su J, Zhang J, Yu L, et al. Real-time swept source optical coherence tomography imaging of the human airway using a microelectromechanical system endoscope and digital signal processor. J Biomed Opt 2008;13:030506:1–3.
31. Qi X, Sivak MV Jr, Isenberg G, et al. Computer-aided diagnosis of dysplasia in Barrett's esophagus using endoscopic optical coherence tomography. J Biomed Opt 2006;11:4–13.
32. Suter M, Vakoc BJ, Yachimski PS, et al. Comprehensive microscopy of the esophagus in human patients with optical frequency domain imaging. Gastrointest Endosc 2008;68:745–53.
33. Wang R, Elder J. Propylene glycol as a contrasting agent for optical coherence tomography to image gastrointestinal tissues. Lasers Surg Med 2002;30:201–8.
34. Testoni P, Mariani A, Mangiavillano B, et al. Intraductal optical coherence tomography for investigating main pancreatic duct strictures. Am J Gastroenterol 2007; 102:269–74.
35. Isenberg G, Pollack MJ, Faulx AL, et al. In vivo imaging of the biliary and pancreatic duct with optical coherence tomography during ERCP accurately identifies dysplastic cellular changes. Gastrointest Endosc 2008;67:AB107.
36. Jeon MY, Zhang J, Wang Q, et al. High-speed and wide bandwidth Fourier domain mode-locked wavelength swept laser with multiple SOAs. Opt Express 2008;16:2547–54.
37. Oh WY, Yun SH, Tearney GJ, et al. Wide tuning range wavelength-swept laser with two semiconductor optical amplifiers. IEEE Photon Tech Lett 2005;17: 678–80.

Confocal Laser Endomicroscopy

Ralf Kiesslich, MD, PhD[a,*], Marcia Irene Canto, MD, MHS[b]

KEYWORDS

- Confocal laser endoscopy • Endomicroscopy • Fluorescence
- Miniprobe • Barrett's esophagus • Gastritis • Gastric cancer
- Celiac disease • Colorectal cancer • Ulcerative colitis

Confocal laser endomicroscopy (CLE) is a new imaging modality for gastrointestinal (GI) endoscopy. It offers in vivo imaging of the mucosal layer at cellular and even subcellular resolution. Thus, in vivo histology becomes possible during ongoing endoscopy. This new imaging modality provides more than conventional histology, because cellular interaction can be observed over time (physiology), and distinct changes can be identified (pathophysiology).

PRINCIPLES OF CONFOCAL MICROSCOPY

Confocal microscopy allows a better spatial resolution compared with that of conventional fluorescence microscopy, because images are not contaminated by light scattering from other focal planes. A low-power laser is focused to a single point in a defined microscopic field of view, and the same lens is used as both condenser and objective folding optical path. Thus, the point of illumination coincides with the point of detection within the specimen. Light emanating from that point is focused through a pinhole to a detector, and light emanating from outside the illuminated spot is rejected from detection. Illumination and detection systems are at the same focal plane and termed as "confocal." All detected signals from the illuminated spot are captured and measured. The created grayscale image is an optical section representing one focal plane within the examined specimen. The image of a scanned region can now be constructed and digitized by measuring light returning to the detector from successive points.

Series of confocal images within successive planes can be used to observe fine (sub)cellular structures, and three-dimensional structures of specimens can also be created. Confocal microscopy has become a standard method for molecular imaging

[a] Department of I. Med. Klinik und Poliklinik, Johannes Gutenberg University, Mainz, Langenbeckstr. 1, 55131 Mainz, Deutschland, Germany
[b] Division of Gastroenterology and Hepatology, Johns Hopkins University School of Medicine, 1830 East Monument Street, Baltimore, MD 21205, USA
* Corresponding author.
E-mail address: info@ralf-kiesslich.de (R. Kiesslich).

Gastrointest Endoscopy Clin N Am 19 (2009) 261–272
doi:10.1016/j.giec.2009.02.007
giendo.theclinics.com
1052-5157/09/$ – see front matter

in basic research in conjunction with fluorescence labeling techniques, thereby permitting the localization of specific proteins at distinct cellular locations. However, confocal microscopy has been mainly performed so far on a microscope stage at the bench rather than the bedside.[1]

ENDOSCOPIC CONFOCAL MICROSCOPY

Endoscopic confocal microscopy is an outgrowth of conventional laboratory confocal microscopy. Currently, two confocal imaging systems are available for in vivo detection of GI diseases: confocal imaging relying on tissue reflectance and confocal imaging based on tissue fluorescence. Reflectance endomicroscopy was first reported by Sakashita and colleagues[2] in 2003. However, reflectance endomicroscopy suffers from poor resolution and contrast.

Fluorescence confocal imaging has overcome these limitations. The first publication about an integrated confocal fluorescence microscope into the distal tip of a conventional colonoscope (Pentax EC 3830FK, Tokyo, Japan) was made in 2004,[3] showing that in vivo microscopy at subcellular resolution (0.7 μm) simultaneously displayed to white light endoscopy became possible and achieved high accuracy. This approach, designated CLE, permitted immediate diagnosis of colorectal intraepithelial neoplasias using fluorescein or acriflavine as contrast agents.

Most recently, a probe-based confocal endomicroscope was developed, which can be passed over the working channel of standard endoscopes. This further miniaturization using fiber-bundle technology results in compromise of resolution: lateral resolution 3.5 μm and axial resolution 15 μm; field of view of 600x500 μm, and fixed imaging plane depth (see **Fig. 1**).[4]

CONTRAST AGENTS

Fluorescence confocal imaging is only possible using exogenous fluorescence contrast agents. Potentially suitable agents are fluorescein, acriflavine, or cresyl violet.[1] The most common contrast agents are acriflavine hydrochloride (0.05% in saline; topical use only) or fluorescein sodium (5–10 mL of a 10% solution; intravenous application). Confocal imaging following staining with acriflavine hydrochloride and fluorescein sodium reveals a characteristic morphology of mucosal tissue. Whereas topically used acriflavine hydrochloride strongly labels the superficial epithelial cells including nuclei, intravenously applied fluorescein sodium distributes throughout the entire mucosa with a strong contrast within the connective tissue and the capillary network. Fluorescein binds to serum albumin, and the remaining, unbound dye molecules pass across systemic capillaries and enter the tissue, highlighting the extracellular matrix. Confocal images can be generated simultaneously with endoscopic images and allow identification of typical histologic structures within the upper and lower GI tract.

CLINICAL APPLICATION OF ENDOMICROSCOPY

Endomicroscopy can be used to observe living cells during ongoing endoscopy. A plethora of changes can be identified by the examiner. Thus, a thorough knowledge about mucosal pathology is mandatory to obtain reliable online diagnosis.

Barrett's Esophagus

Barrett's esophagus is known to be a premalignant condition in patients with gastroesophageal reflux disease, and most adenocarcinomas of the distal esophagus have

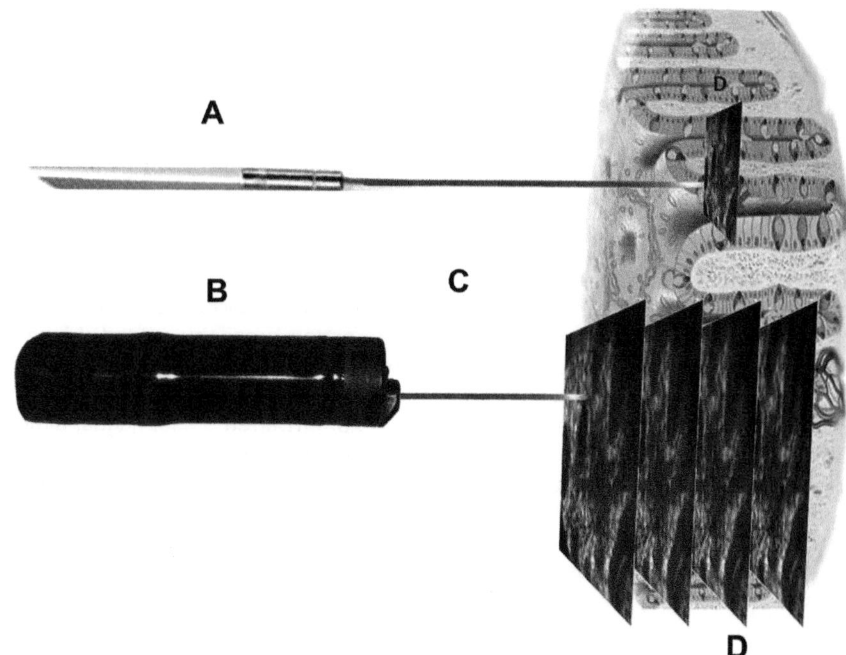

Fig. 1. Types of confocal endomicroscopy. Two different confocal endomicroscopic systems are currently available. The miniprobe (*A*) can be passed over the working channel of standard endoscopes (MaunaKea, France). (*B*) The endomicroscope is embedded in an otherwise standard endoscope (Pentax, Japan). The blue laser light is applied onto and into the mucosa (*C*). The fluorescence and reflected light are measured, and grey scale images of mucosal microarchitecture are displayed on an additional monitor. The miniprobe has a fixed imaging plane depth (*D*), whereas the confocal endoscope can vary the imaging-plane depth during imaging from the surface up to the deepest parts of the mucosal layer.

been shown to arise in Barrett's tissue. Barrett's esophagus is defined histologically by the presence of specialized columnar epithelium (SCE) with goblet cells. The columnar-lined lower esophagus (CLE) can be identified during standard upper endoscopy. SCE is often present in a patchy mosaic contribution within CLE and can be overlooked by random biopsies, resulting in biopsies of the cardia or gastric type of mucosa without goblet cells. However, it has been suggested that 4-quadrant step biopsies within CLE should serve as the gold standard for diagnosing Barrett's epithelium and Barrett's-associated neoplastic changes.

Endomicroscopy makes it possible to identify CLE macroscopically and identify goblet cells microscopically in the distal esophagus, allowing an immediate and reliable diagnosis of Barrett's esophagus. In the first endomicroscopic study on Barrett's esophagus with 63 patients, different types of epithelial cells could be distinguished, and cellular and vascular changes were detected using fluorescein-guided endomicroscopy.[5] A classification of confocal images for the diagnosis of Barrett's epithelium and Barrett's-associated neoplasias was developed on the basis of a comparison of the in vivo and conventional ex vivo histology. The classification distinguishes between three types of epithelium (gastric epithelium; Barrett's epithelium without neoplastic changes; and Barrett's epithelium with neoplastic changes).

In the first study dealing with endomicroscopy in patients with Barrett's esophagus,[5] 156 areas and 3012 images were retrospectively reviewed in accordance with the newly developed Confocal Barrett Classification and compared with the pathologic examination of targeted mucosal biopsies (411 biopsies). The comparison showed that Barrett's esophagus could be predicted by confocal endomicroscopy based on the identification of goblet cells, with a sensitivity of 98.1% and a specificity of 94.1%, respectively (accuracy, 96.8%; positive predictive value, 97.2%; negative predictive value, 96.0%). Moreover, Barrett's-associated neoplastic changes could be predicted based on irregular black cells with a sensitivity of 92.9% and a specificity of 98.4%, respectively (accuracy, 97.4%; positive predictive value, 92.9%; negative predictive value, 98.4%) (see **Fig. 2**).

This first study was subsequently confirmed prospectively in a randomized crossover design comparing standard endoscopy with random biopsy and endomicroscopy with targeted biopsy.[6] In this study, endomicroscopy-guided biopsies improved the yield for detection of neoplasia from 17% to 33% in a group of patients with suspected nonlocalized endoscopically inapparent high-grade dysplasia (n = 16). In patients undergoing routine surveillance (n = 23) of Barrett's esophagus, almost two-thirds were able to forgo mucosal biopsies, as no neoplasia was found to be present during endomicroscopic imaging. Thus, confocal endomicroscopy (Pentax system) with targeted biopsy can allow the endoscopist to take smarter biopsies and could potentially reduce the delay to definitive therapy in patients with Barrett's-associated neoplasia.[6] Furthermore, endomicroscopy is able to guide mucosal resection.[7]

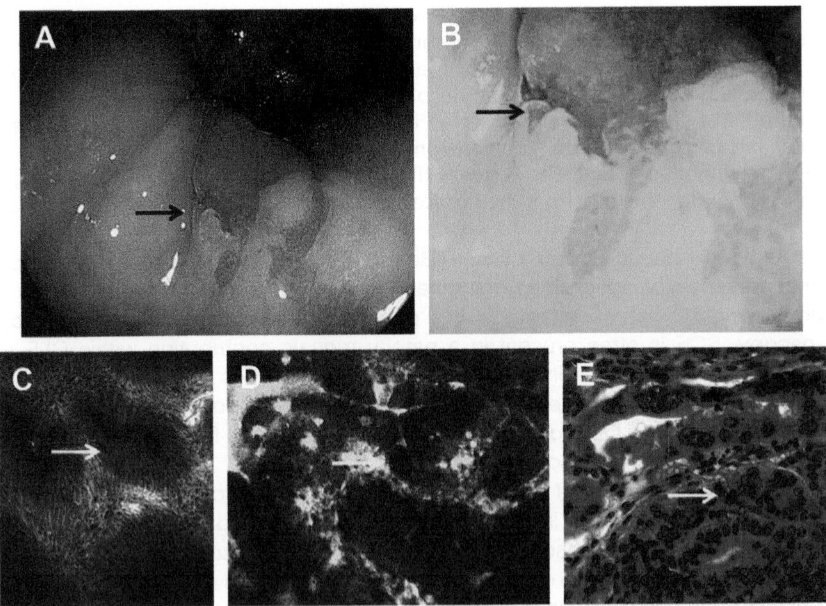

Fig. 2. Confocal endomicroscopy of early Barrett's cancer. (*A*) Short Barrett's esophagus is visible with white light endoscopy. A subtle depression can be identified (*arrow*). (*B*) I-Scan function (postprocessing light filter) helps to highlight the subtle changes. (*C*) Normal, non-neoplastic Barrett glands are characterized by their roundish appearance and their presence of goblet cells (*arrow*). (*D*) Malignant cellular architectures are characterized by dark irregular cells with different shapes and sizes (*arrow*). The infiltration of malignant cells into the lamina propria can be observed, defining at least mucosal cancer. (*E*) Endomicroscopic-guided mucosal resection revealed early Barrett's cancer (ms; well differentiated).

Most recently, 2008 data are also available for the miniprobe-based confocal microscopy.[8]

About 296 biopsy sites in 38 consecutive patients with Barrett's esophagus were examined with standard high-resolution endoscopy and by miniprobe endomicroscopy. Endomicroscopy examined areas were matched with biopsies using argon plasma coagulation marking of the examined tissue. The criteria for Barrett's esophagus and associated neoplasia were established based on 15 patients, and these criteria were prospectively investigated in 23 patients using video recording of the endomicroscopic examination.

In a per-biopsy analysis, sensitivity and specificity for the two independent investigators were 75.0% and 88.8% and 75.0% and 91.0%, respectively, translating at best into a positive predictive value of 44.4% and a negative predictive value of 98.8%. Interobserver agreement was good (kappa 0.6). The diagnostic yield of miniprobe-based endomicroscopy seems to be lower than that of the integrated-type endomicroscopy, which might be a result of the lower resolution and the fixed imaging-plane depth of the confocal miniprobe.

Gastritis and Gastric Cancer

Gastritis is defined histologically by various stages of inflammatory changes. These include infiltration of inflammatory cells into the lamina propria, often combined with alteration and defects of the mucosal surface, such as erosions. *Helicobacter pylori* or nonsteroidal anti-inflammatory drugs can induce gastritis. The former can lead to atrophic gastritis and intestinal metaplasia, which increase the risk for the development of gastric cancer.

H pylori and intestinal metaplasia can be easily identified using CLE.[9–11] *H pylori* can be found on the surface of the gastric mucosa. Thus, acriflavine as a topical contrast agent has to be used to identify *H pylori*. Intestinal metaplasia can be best seen using fluorescein. The tissue looks much brighter compared with the surrounding normal mucosa, and characteristic goblet cells can be identified due to their characteristic target phenomenon (see **Fig. 3**). Endomicroscopy is ideally suited to diagnose

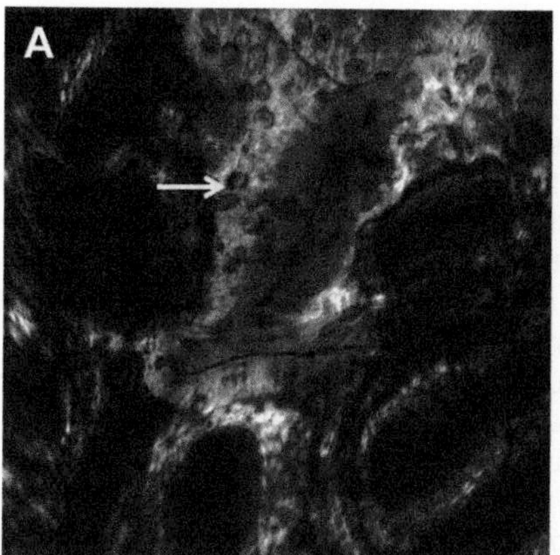

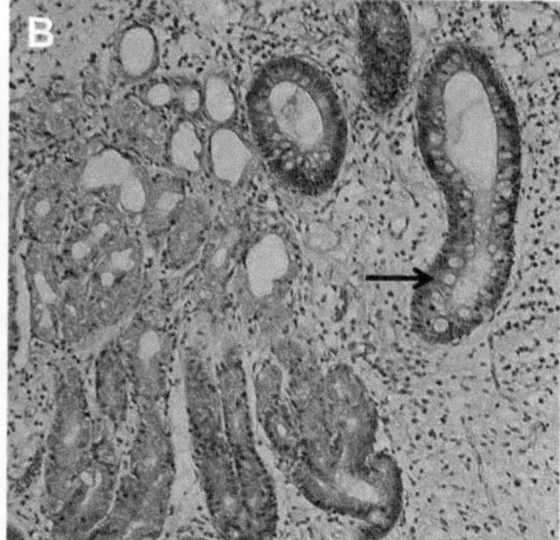

Fig. 3. Atrophic gastritis and intestinal metaplasia of the stomach. (*A*) The different tissue components (normal gastric mucosa and intestinal metaplasia) are readily identified due to their distinct staining patterns. Intestinal metaplasia is characterized by a brighter aspect with the presence of goblet cells (*arrow*). (*B*) Endomicroscopic-guided biopsies confirmed the presence of intestinal metaplasia and atrophic gastritis.

intestinal metaplasia in patients with atrophic gastritis. Furthermore, *H pylori* can be identified in vivo, and distinct cellular and vascular changes guide biopsies toward neoplastic changes.

The endoscopic detection of early gastric cancer is challenging, because most of the lesions are usually nonpolypoid. Fluorescein-guided endomicroscopy is particularly good at demonstrating blood vessel architecture, which can be used to differentiate between non-neoplastic and neoplastic lesions. The vessel function can be observed, and leakage of fluorescein into the lamina propria characterizes inflammation or neoangiogenesis.[12] Endomicroscopy allows immediate microscopic analysis of the gastric mucosa during ongoing endoscopy. Comparison of regular and altered gastric mucosa facilitates the interpretation of the confocal images. Changes in tissue and microscopic blood vessel architecture as well as changes in cell morphology are valuable endomicroscopic criteria to define neoplasia. Nuclear changes can best be observed using acriflavine as topical contrast agent as shown by Kakeji and colleagues.[13]

Zhang and colleagues[10] investigated the pattern and in vivo architecture of gastritis and gastric cancer on 132 consecutive patients. The confocal images obtained from the 132 patients were compared with the histopathologic findings of the biopsy specimens from the corresponding confocal imaging sites in a prospective and blinded fashion. Gastric pit-pattern cellular architecture was classified into seven types. Normal mucosa with fundic glands mainly showed type A (round pits), and corporal mucosa with histologic gastritis showed type B (noncontinuous short rod-like); normal mucosa with pyloric glands mainly showed type C (continuous short rod-like), and antral mucosa with histologic gastritis showed type D (elongated and tortuous branch-like). Goblet cells could be easily identified by confocal endomicroscopy in intestinal metaplasia mucosa, which showed type E. The sensitivity and specificity of the type E pattern for predicting gastric atrophy were 83.6% and 99.6%, respectively. Corresponding values of the type G pattern for predicting gastric cancer were 90.0% and 99.4%.

Kitabatake and colleagues were able to show differences of mucosal vasculature according to the grade of tumor differentiation using endomicroscopy. The accuracy for the diagnosis of gastric cancer using endomicroscopy was above 90% if a good image quality was provided.[14]

Celiac Disease

Celiac disease (CD) is very common in western countries; it is associated with a risk of malignant transformation and severe illness due to malabsorption. Current endoscopic techniques cannot diagnose CD as accurately as histopathology. Most recently, the value of endomicroscopy in patients with CD was evaluated and showed promising results.[15] Subjects with CD and controls were prospectively studied with endomicroscopy using fluorescein as contrast agent. Features of villous atrophy and crypt hypertrophy were defined by endomicroscopy. The newly developed score measuring CD severity in vivo was devised and validated against the diagnosis of CD and blinded histopathology. Receiver-operator characteristics, sensitivity to change after treatment, and reliability of findings were assessed. From 31 patients (six untreated CD, 11 treated CD, and 14 controls), 7019 confocal endomicroscopy (CEM) images paired with 326 biopsy specimens were obtained. The accuracy of CEM in diagnosing CD was excellent (receiver-operator characteristics area under the curve, 0.946; sensitivity, 94%; specificity, 92%) and correlated well with the Marsh grading (R-squared, 0.756). CEM differentiated CD from controls ($P < .0001$) and was sensitive to change after treatment with gluten-free diet (1787 optical biopsies;

$P = .012$). The intraclass correlation of reliability was high (0.759–0.916). Of the 17 cases with diagnosed CD, 16 (94%) were diagnosed correctly using CEM, but only 13 (76%) had detectable histopathology changes. The procedure was safe and well tolerated. Thus, endomicroscopy has a great potential to improve endoscopy efficiency and clinical algorithm in patients with CD.

Colorectal Cancer

Colorectal cancer is still one of the leading causes of cancer-related death in the western world. Screening colonoscopy is widely accepted as the gold standard for early diagnosis of cancer. The prognosis for patients with colonic neoplasm is strictly dependent on the depth of infiltration, and, therefore, depends on early detection of preinvasive and neoplastic changes. Early detection makes it possible to cure the patient by immediate endoscopic resection.

In 2003, Inoue and colleagues[16] reported initial experience with real-time, ultrahigh magnification endoscopy in ex vivo specimens. The prototype endocytoscope that was used (Olympus Optical Ltd., Tokyo, Japan) was passed through the working channel of an endoscope. The aim of the study was to establish new criteria for distinguishing between benign lesions and high-grade dysplasia or cancer. The authors examined 100 endoscopically or surgically visualized normal colonic mucosa or hyperplastic polyps, but they were more often visible in neoplastic lesions. Conversely, goblet cells were visible less often in malignant or premalignant lesions. However, it should be noted that it was not individual nuclei but rather dark areas in irregular cells that were visible. The study found a statistically significant difference between non-neoplastic and neoplastic lesions in relation to the detection rate of nuclei (dark areas) in laser-scanning confocal microscopy images. On the basis of these results, the authors recommended preliminary criteria for an endoscopic microscopic cytologic imaging classification of high-grade intraepithelial neoplasia and cancer. Neoplasia was characterized by the presence of any structural abnormality and clear visualization of nuclei. However, the sensitivity of this method for predicting neoplasia in the colorectum was only 60%, reflecting the limited resolution of the system that was used.

In contrast to endocytoscopy, which images the most superficial epithelial cells at a fixed depth, endomicroscopy can visualize both mucosal cell and blood vessel abnormalities. In the first study using the newly developed endomicroscopic system, 42 patients with indications for screening or surveillance colonoscopy after previous polypectomy underwent in vivo endomicroscopy with the confocal laser endoscope.[3] The aim of the study was to assess the histology in vivo during ongoing colonoscopy to diagnose intraepithelial neoplasias or colon cancer. Fluorescein-guided endomicroscopy of intraepithelial neoplasias and colon cancers showed a tubular, villous, or irregular architecture, with a reduced number of goblet cells. In addition, neovascularization in neoplasms was characterized by irregular vessel architecture with fluorescein leakage.

A simple classification of the confocal pattern, based on initial experience with confocal endomicroscopy, was developed to allow differentiation between neoplastic and non-neoplastic tissue. Macroscopic and microscopic images were taken together to allow an immediate prediction of the histopathology. A total of 13,020 confocal images from 390 locations were compared with the histological data from 1038 biopsies. It was possible to predict the presence of neoplastic changes using the newly developed confocal pattern classification, with a sensitivity of 97.4%, a specificity of 99.4%, and an accuracy of 99.2%, respectively (see **Fig. 4**).[3]

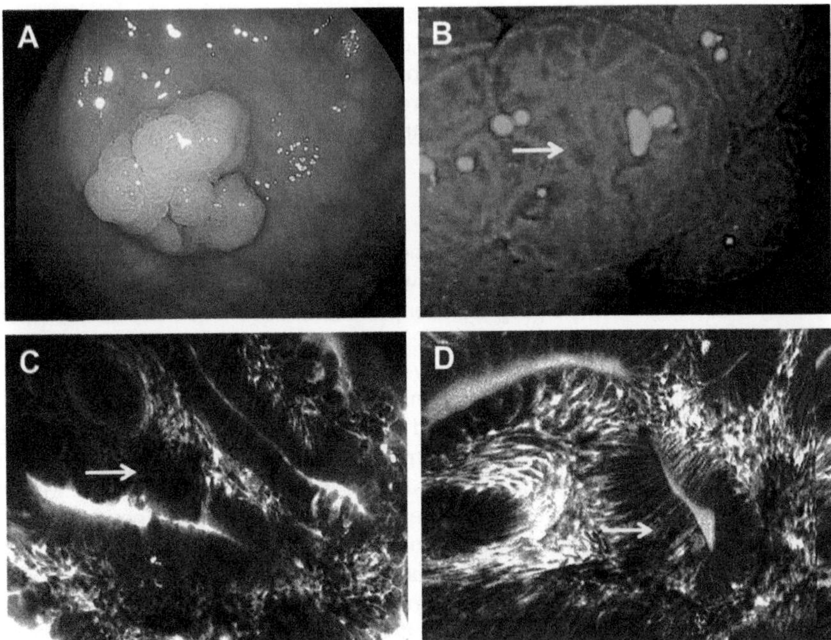

Fig. 4. Tubulovillous adenoma of the rectum. (*A*) A flat adenoma is present in the sigmoid. (*B*) Close observation using magnifying endoscopy unmasks the surface staining pattern (Kudo's classification III L). Epithelial cell bands can be identified (*arrow*). (*C*) Endomicroscopy confirms the presence of tubular adenoma. The tubular architecture as well as single cells can be identified (*arrow*). (*D*) Depletion of goblet cells indicates the presence of intraepithelial neoplasia (*arrow*).

Ulcerative Colitis

It is not possible to examine the whole surface of the colon in the endomicroscopic mode. In patients with ulcerative colitis, it is, therefore, important to combine endomicroscopy with chromoendoscopy. Panchromoendoscopy with either methylene blue or indigo carmine is a valid diagnostic tool for improving the diagnostic yield of intraepithelial neoplasia using the "SURFACE" recommendations.[17] Chromoendoscopy can reveal circumscribed lesions, and chromoendoscopic-guided CLE can be used to predict intraepithelial neoplasias with a high degree of accuracy.[18] Targeted biopsies of relevant lesions can, therefore, be taken, and rapid confirmation of neoplastic changes using confocal laser endoscopy during colonoscopy may lead to significant improvements in the clinical management.

In the first randomized trial of endomicroscopy in ulcerative colitis, 153 patients with long-term ulcerative colitis who were in clinical remission were randomly assigned at a ratio of 1:1 to undergo either conventional colonoscopy or panchromoendoscopy using 0.1% methylene blue in conjunction with endomicroscopy to detect intraepithelial neoplasia or colorectal cancer.[18] Circumscribed lesions in the colonic mucosa detected by chromoendoscopy were evaluated with endomicroscopy for cellular and vascular changes in accordance with the confocal pattern classification for predicting neoplasia. Targeted biopsies from the areas examined were taken and histologically graded according to the New Vienna classification.

In the standard colonoscopy group, randomized biopsies every 10 cm between the anus and cecum were taken, as along with targeted biopsies of visible mucosal changes. The primary outcome analysis was a histological diagnosis of neoplasia. Using chromoendoscopy in conjunction with endomicroscopy (80 patients; average examination time, 42 minutes), significantly more intraepithelial neoplasia was detected (19 vs 4 cases; $P = .007$) compared to standard colonoscopy (73 patients; average examination time, 31 minutes). Endomicroscopy revealed different cellular structures (epithelial and blood cells), capillaries, and connective tissue limited to the mucosal layer. A total of 5580 confocal images from 134 circumscribed lesions were compared with the histological results from 311 biopsies. The presence of neoplastic changes was predicted with a high degree of accuracy (sensitivity, 94.7%; specificity, 98.3%; accuracy 97.8%).[18]

In summary, chromoendoscopy is able to reveal circumscribed colonic mucosal neoplastic lesions, and confocal laser microscopy can be used to confirm intraepithelial neoplasias with a high degree of accuracy. Biopsies can, therefore, be limited to targeted sampling of relevant lesions. In vivo histology with endomicroscopy may lead to significant improvements in the clinical management of patients with ulcerative colitis, with reduced numbers of biopsies being needed for confirmation of the condition and time being gained for immediate therapeutic intervention.

Microscopic Colitis

Microscopic colitis is a term used to define clinicopathologic entities characterized by chronic watery diarrhea, normal radiological and endoscopic appearances, and microscopic abnormalities. Specific histopathological appearances can be used to further classify collagenous colitis, lymphocytic colitis, and other conditions. Collagenous colitis differs from lymphocytic colitis by the presence of a subepithelial collagen band (≥ 10 μm) adjacent to the basal membrane. Both diseases disclose inflammatory changes in the lamina propria and superficial epithelial damage. Although microscopic colitis is considered a rare condition, increasing awareness of these entities among pathologists and clinicians has resulted in more frequent diagnosis. However, their incidence is not well known. However, the incidence of lymphocytic colitis is about three times higher than that of collagenous colitis, and microscopic colitis should be considered as a major possibility in the workup of chronic diarrhea in older women.

Endomicroscopy makes it possible to locate and measure the distribution and thickness of collagenous bands underneath the epithelial layer, thus allowing targeted biopsies. This is a new approach in collagenous colitis, particularly in cases with disrupted subepithelial collagen deposits. At present, randomized biopsies are recommended, preferably from the right colon. The distribution of the collagenous bands can be patchy and segmental in the colon. Confocal endomicroscopy helps differentiate between affected and normal sites and can guide biopsies.[19,20]

FUTURE OF ENDOMICROSCOPY

Endomicroscopy cannot be used only to receive histology. The great potential of endomicroscopy is to display and observe physiologic and pathophysiologic changes during ongoing endoscopy. Furthermore, molecular imaging becomes possible.

Cell shedding is a physiologic process. After cell shedding, an epithelial gap occurs; this is sealed within seconds. Patients with inflammatory bowel disease show malfunction of gap closure, which can lead to invasion of bacteria into the lamina propria (see **Fig. 5**). These changes can be observed with endomicroscopy and might define new options for the treatment of inflammatory bowel diseases.[21] Endomicroscopy displays not only tissue but also bacterial interaction with the mucosal layer.[22]

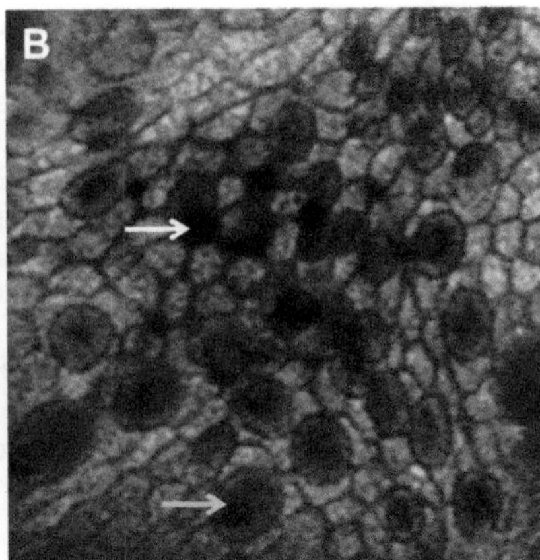

Fig. 5. Differentiation of goblet cells and epithelial gaps. (*A*) Healthy colonic mucosa is seen using acriflavine-aided endomicroscopy. Single round crypts are present. Epithelial gaps are present after cell shedding (*square*). (*B*) Further magnification shows the difference between gaps (*yellow arrow*) and goblet cells (*blue arrow*). Goblet cells have a distinct target sign, whereas gaps are displayed as completely black roundish areas.

Molecular imaging has already been achieved.[23] Dysplastic colonic crypts could be selectively stained with heptapeptides, which were linked with fluorescein. This approach will open the door for new clinical algorithms, which will be dependent on the endomicroscopic findings (eg, prediction of the efficiency of chemotherapy with biologicals).

The diagnostic spectrum of endomicroscopy is constantly increasing, and the borders of the GI tract have already been passed. Endomicroscopy can be used to investigate the bile duct, liver, and cervix.[24–26]

SUMMARY

Endomicroscopy is a revolutionary technique that has significantly broadened the diagnostic spectrum of GI endoscopy. It provides in vivo histology, which is currently mainly used to guide biopsy. However, endomicroscopy will be additionally used to better understand physiology and pathophysiology, which will lead to new diagnostic algorithms that are based on newly discovered microscopic alterations of the mucosal layer. The possibilities of endomicroscopy are extensive, and we have just started to discover them. Thus, endomicroscopy will be a crucial part of the endoscopist's armamentarium of the future.

REFERENCES

1. Atlas of Endomicroscopy. In: Kiesslich R, Galle PR, Neurath MF, editors. Germany: Springer; 2008.
2. Sakashita M, Inoue H, Kashida H, et al. Virtual histology of colorectal lesions using laser-scanning confocal microscopy. Endoscopy 2003;35(12):1033–8.
3. Kiesslich R, Burg J, Vieth M, et al. Confocal laser endoscopy for diagnosing intraepithelial neoplasias and colorectal cancer in vivo. Gastroenterology 2004;127(3):706–13.

4. Meining A, Saur D, Bajbouj M, et al. In vivo histopathology for detection of gastrointestinal neoplasia with a portable, confocal miniprobe: an examiner blinded analysis. Clin Gastroenterol Hepatol 2007;5(11):1261–7.
5. Kiesslich R, Gossner L, Goetz M, et al. In vivo histology of Barrett's esophagus and associated neoplasia by confocal laser endomicroscopy. Clin Gastroenterol Hepatol 2006;4(8):979–87.
6. Dunbar K, Okolo P, Montgomery E, et al. Confocal Endomicroscopy in Barrett's Esophagus and Endoscopically Inapparent Barrett's Neoplasia: A Prospective Randomized Double-Blind Controlled Crossover Trial. Gastrointest Endosc, in press.
7. Leung KK, Maru D, Abraham S, et al. Optical EMR: confocal endomicroscopy-targeted EMR of focal high-grade dysplasia in Barrett's esophagus. Gastrointest Endosc 2008, in press.
8. Pohl H, Rösch T, Vieth M, et al. Miniprobe confocal laser microscopy for the detection of invisible neoplasia in patients with Barrett's oesophagus. Gut 2008; 57(12):1648–53.
9. Guo YT, Li YQ, Yu T, et al. Diagnosis of gastric intestinal metaplasia with confocal laser endomicroscopy in vivo: a prospective study. Endoscopy 2008;40(7): 547–53.
10. Zhang JN, Li YQ, Zhao YA, et al. Classification of gastric pit patterns by confocal endomicroscopy. Gastrointest Endosc 2008;67(6):843–53.
11. Kiesslich R, Goetz M, Burg J, et al. Diagnosing *Helicobacter pylori* in vivo by confocal laser endoscopy. Gastroenterology 2005;128(7):2119–23.
12. Liu H, Li YQ, Yu T, et al. Confocal endomicroscopy for in vivo detection of microvascular architecture in normal and malignant lesions of upper gastrointestinal tract. J Gastroenterol Hepatol 2008;23(1):56–61.
13. Kakeji Y, Yamaguchi S, Yoshida D, et al. Development and assessment of morphologic criteria for diagnosing gastric cancer using confocal endomicroscopy: an ex vivo and in vivo study. Endoscopy 2006;38(9):886–90.
14. Kitabatake S, Niwa Y, Miyahara R, et al. Confocal endomicroscopy for the diagnosis of gastric cancer in vivo. Endoscopy 2006;38(11):1110–4.
15. Leong RW, Nguyen NQ, Meredith CG, et al. In vivo confocal endomicroscopy in the diagnosis and evaluation of celiac disease. Gastroenterology 2008;135(6): 1870–6.
16. Inoue H, Cho JY, Satodate H, et al. Development of virtual histology and virtual biopsy using laser-scanning confocal microscopy. Scand J Gastroenterol Suppl 2003;(237):37–9.
17. Kiesslich R, Neurath MF. Surveillance colonoscopy in ulcerative colitis: magnifying chromoendoscopy in the spotlight. Gut 2004;53(2):165–7.
18. Kiesslich R, Goetz M, Lammersdorf K, et al. Chromoscopy-guided endomicroscopy increases the diagnostic yield of intraepithelial neoplasia in ulcerative colitis. Gastroenterology 2007;132(3):874–82.
19. Kiesslich R, Hoffman A, Goetz M, et al. In vivo diagnosis of collagenous colitis by confocal endomicroscopy. Gut 2006;55(4):591–2.
20. Zambelli A, Villanacci V, Buscarini E, et al. Collagenous colitis: a case series with confocal laser microscopy and histology correlation. Endoscopy 2008;40(7):606–8.
21. Kiesslich R, Goetz M, Angus EM, et al. Identification of epithelial gaps in human small and large intestine by confocal endomicroscopy. Gastroenterology 2007; 133(6):1769–78.
22. Günther U, Epple HJ, Heller F, et al. In vivo diagnosis of intestinal spirochaetosis by confocal endomicroscopy. Gut 2008;57(9):1331–3.

23. Hsiung PL, Hardy J, Friedland S, et al. Detection of colonic dysplasia in vivo using a targeted heptapeptide and confocal microendoscopy. Nat Med 2008;14(4): 454–8.
24. Meining A, Frimberger E, Becker V, et al. Detection of cholangiocarcinoma in vivo using miniprobe-based confocal fluorescence microscopy. Clin Gastroenterol Hepatol 2008;6(9):1057–60.
25. Goetz M, Kiesslich R, Dienes HP, et al. In vivo confocal laser endomicroscopy of the human liver: a novel method for assessing liver microarchitecture in real time. Endoscopy 2008;40(7):554–62.
26. Tan J, Delaney P. Confocal endomicroscopy: a novel imaging technique for in vivo histology of cervical intraepithelial neoplasia. Expert Rev Med Devices 2007;4(6):863–71.

Endocytoscopy in Esophageal Cancer

Yutaka Tomizawa, MD, Hamza M. Abdulla, Ganapathy A. Prasad, MD, Louis-Michel Wong Kee Song, MD, Lori S. Lutzke, CCRP, Lynn S. Borkenhagen, RN, Kenneth K. Wang, MD*

KEYWORDS

- Esophagectomy • Photodynamic therapy
- Endoscopic mucosal resection • Barrett's esophagus
- Esophageal carcinoma • Outcomes • Recurrence

The ability to visualize in vivo microscopic areas of neoplasia within gastrointestinal mucosa has been a major quest of modern gastroenterology. The attainment of this goal could revolutionize the diagnosis and treatment of neoplastic disease. Potential benefits could include the elimination of random biopsies for surveillance of mucosal disease, increasing time intervals between surveillance endoscopy, elimination of sampling error issues, decrease in interprocedural discrepancies regarding the presence and magnitude of dysplasia present, and ultimately improving patient outcomes with at-risk neoplasia. Recent advances in endocytoscopy can help guide the early detection of malignancy and lead to earlier treatment. Endocytoscopy is a new imaging and magnification technology classified as one of the "contact devices" and has been developed for observation of cellular structure in vivo with particular application in the esophagus. The technology can provide accurate targeting of lesions with an in vivo "virtual histologic diagnosis" and could enhance endoscopic surveillance by decreasing biopsies of normal-appearing mucosa. The purpose of this review is to survey the technology available and examine the literature to date regarding its clinical usage. We also conclude this review with potential future directions.

Esophageal cancer has one of the highest cancer mortality rates in the Unites States. It is estimated that there will be 16,470 new patients diagnosed with esophageal cancer and 14,280 deaths from it in 2008.[1] Rapidly increasing incidence of esophageal adenocarcinoma, especially among white men, has been reported in the United States, although squamous cell carcinoma of the esophagus has been

---

Supported by NIH grants: R01CA111603-01A1 (KKW), R01CA097048 (KKW), R21CA122426-01 (KKW) and the Shirley and Miles Fiterman Digestive Disease Center.

Barrett's Esophagus Unit, Division of Gastroenterology and Hepatology, St.Mary's Hospital, Mayo Clinic College of Medicine, Alfred Main, 200, 1st Street SW, Rochester, MN 55905, USA
* Corresponding author.
E-mail address: wang.kenneth@mayo.edu (K.K. Wang).

Gastrointest Endoscopy Clin N Am 19 (2009) 273–281
doi:10.1016/j.giec.2009.02.006 **giendo.theclinics.com**
1052-5157/09/$ – see front matter

declining in recent decades. In fact, a report in 2008 shows that esophageal adenocarcinoma incidence rates rose from 1975 through 2004 among white men and women in all stages and age groups. The incidence of esophageal adenocarcinoma among white men increased 463%, from 1.01 per 100,000 person years in 1975 to 1979 to 5.69 per 100,000 person years in 2000 to 2004. A similar rapid increase was also apparent among white women, with an increased incident of 335% from 0.17 per 100,000 person years to 0.74 person years.[2] This increase was not clear in earlier reports because of the rarity of esophageal adenocarcinoma among women. Recent data indicate that the incidence of esophageal adenocarcinoma is a growing health problem for white Americans. The known risk factors for esophageal adenocarcinoma are chronic gastroesophageal reflux disease and Barrett's esophagus.[3] Persons with recurring symptoms of reflux have an eight-fold increase in the risk of esophageal adenocarcinoma.[4] Among patients with Barrett's esophagus, the annual rate of neoplastic transformation is reported to be approximately 0.5%.[5]

BARRETT'S ESOPHAGUS AND ESOPHAGEAL ADENOCARCINOMA

Barrett's esophagus is a condition in which the normal squamous epithelium of the esophagus is replaced by metaplastic columnar mucosa. This phenomenon is a complication of esophageal mucosal damage caused by gastroesophageal reflux disease.

It is thought that histologic intestinal metaplasia in Barrett's esophagus progresses sequentially and at a relatively slow pace from no dysplasia to low-grade dysplasia, then to high-grade dysplasia, and eventually to esophageal adenocarcinoma. Although Barrett's esophagus is recognized as a premalignant lesion that may progress to esophageal adenocarcinoma, it does not produce any symptoms. Another factor to consider is the dismal prognosis of esophageal adenocarcinoma (**Fig. 1**). Because the esophagus receives lymphatic supply into the lamina propria, lymph node metastasis is common even in early disease. The prognosis of esophageal adenocarcinoma is dependent on the stage of the disease. Early neoplastic lesions have an excellent prognosis, and the prognosis of most advanced lesions is dismal. Therefore, we should focus on early recognition of Barrett's esophagus and

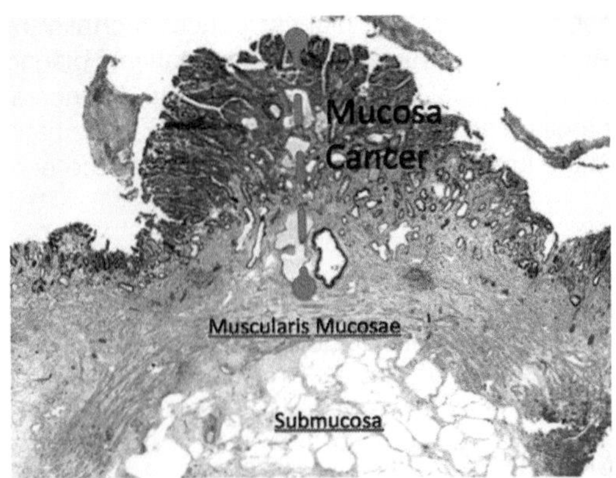

Fig. 1. Esophageal mucosa. This is an image of an early esophageal cancer. The muscularis mucosae is intact, indicating that this is a T1a or early stage cancer. Once there is penetration into the submucosa, the risk of metastatic disease increases significantly.

continuous surveillance for esophageal adenocarcinoma among patients of Barrett's esophagus.

The goal of surveillance is to diagnose early stages of esophageal adenocarcinoma in patients with known Barrett's esophagus and to intervene so as to prevent progression to fatal cancer.[6]

The current recommendations for management of Barrett's esophagus are based on updated guidelines by the Practice Parameters Committee of the American College of Gastroenterology.[7] This guideline consists of two distinct components, screening and surveillance. The diagnosis of Barrett's esophagus should be made only with endoscopy and biopsy of columnar-lined esophagus. Histologic changes in intestinal metaplasia (goblet cells) are needed for the diagnosis before recommendations for surveillance. Once we enroll patients with Barrett's esophagus in a surveillance program, most of the surveillance has been done with endoscopies until now. Four quadrant biopsies every 2 cm of the Barrett's mucosa are recommended to recognize the evidence of dysplasia in the Barrett's mucosa. In addition, the grade of dysplasia determines the appropriate surveillance interval. The more advanced the disease in terms of dysplasia, the more frequently surveillance is needed. Although histologic evidence of metaplasia for diagnosis and evidence of dysplasia for surveillance are currently used, these programs are problematic. There are issues with sampling errors, interobserver interpretation variability between endoscopists,[8] and need for frequent endoscopies. Although sampling errors are minimized by a very vigorous biopsy protocol, such a protocol is unrealistic in general practice, and difficulty to follow makes a low compliance. The purpose of management of Barrett's esophagus is to diagnose malignancy at an early stage and to prevent advanced lesion rate. In terms of detecting malignancy, any nodular areas within the Barrett's segment, especially if high-grade dysplasia has previously been found, are associated with a higher frequency of malignancy.[9] However, occult malignancy may still be present in spite of careful endoscopic surveillance. Lacking mucosal abnormalities and malignancy under normal esophageal mucosa are likely causes in such cases.

Though Barrett's esophagus is an excellent target for optical imaging strategies such as endocytoscopy, this technology can be applied to several different organ systems, including the colon and the biliary system. The problems are similar, although factors such as the limited length of Barrett's esophagus help with the use of imaging devices in this condition. In addition, ease of access and the relative cleanness of the mucosa are also advantages.

ENDOCYTOSCOPY

In recent years, new techniques have been introduced to improve endoscopic recognition of abnormal lesions within Barrett's esophagus. Since the esophagus is easily accessible using endoscopy and the length of required observation is limited, many different types of new optical modalities have been attempted, and they show promising data. Those different techniques can be divided into two categories depending on the purposes.[10] The first one is for primary detection of lesion using imaging of the entire mucosal surface (eg, high-resolution endoscopy, chromoendoscopy, and autofluorescence imaging). The second is for the point inspection of Barrett's lesions after primary detection (eg, spectroscopic devices, optical coherence tomography). Endocytoscopy, though it involves a miniendoscope, falls into the second of these categories.

Endocytoscopy is based on the technology of light-contact microscopy. This imaging tool was first introduced in the field of otolaryngology. After application of methylene blue stain, the surface epithelium with light-contact endoscopy was visible, and cytologic details of the vocal cord were directly visualized during observation.[11,12] However, the endoscopic system used in these studies was a rigid instrument, which is not practical for the gastrointestinal tract. A novel endocytoscopy system is available and termed the Endocytoscope (Prototype, Olympus Medical Systems Corp., Tokyo, Japan). Prototype one gives a low magnification (XEC300) with a maximal 450x magnification and a field of view covering a 300 × 300 μm. Prototype two provides a high magnification (XEC120) with a maximal 1100x magnification and a field of view covering a 120 × 120 μm. The outer diameter of the endoscope is 3.4 mm, which can pass through a working channel with a diameter of 3.7 mm of a mother endoscope (**Fig. 2**).

This usually requires a therapeutic endoscope. Recently, this new imaging modality has been used for observation of the in vivo mucosal surface of the gastrointestinal tract.[13,14] Kumagai and colleagues[15] reported the in vivo application of contact endocytoscopy to 12 patients with superficial esophageal squamous cell carcinoma. In this initial study, approximately 10 mL of 1% methylene blue stain was applied to the mucosa before the procedure. The mucosa also must be cleaned of any mucous to allow uptake of the dye. Usually, this is done using a low concentration of N-acetylcysteine at a dilute concentration such as 1%. Using the low-power magnifying endoscope (XEC-300), the image showed that the density of the cells in all of the cancer lesions was much higher than that of the normal squamous lesions. Using the high-power magnifying endoscope, irregularities in cell distribution, extreme heterogeneity of the cells with the nuclei showing different staining, size and shape characteristics, as well as an irregular nucleus/cytoplasm ratio were visualized. Inoue and colleagues[16] reported applying endocytoscopy to the gastrointestinal tract of 87 patients at the same period. In their study, high-quality images were acquired in 83 cases (95.4%), and insufficient images of four cases were stomach lesions in which gastric mucous secretions prevented clear staining of the nucleus with methylene blue. In these two initial studies, a catheter-based endoscopy system, in which a prototype endocytoscope was passed through into the working channel of the mother endoscope with a short transparent distance cap, was placed at the distal end of the endsocope. A different study introduced a new endocytoscope, which

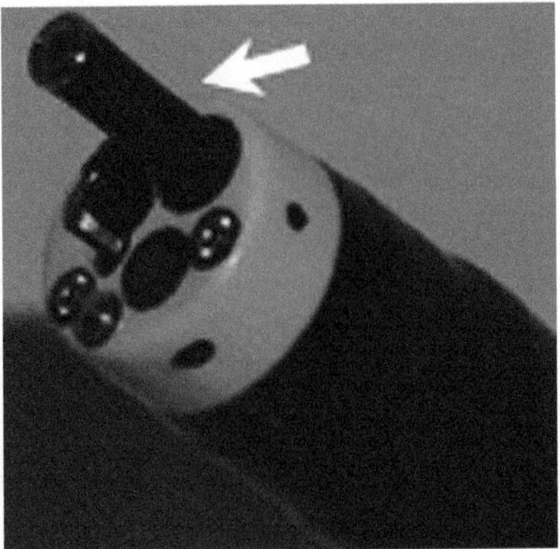

Fig. 2. Endocytoscopy instrument in the channel of a therapeutic endoscope (*arrow*).

was integrated into a regular endoscope with substantial extending imaging spectrum.[17] The new prototype, upper-gastrointestinal instrument (Olympus XGIF-Q260EC1, Olympus Medical Systems Corp) includes a conventional video endoscope with low-power magnification (maximum 80x) and a high-power magnifying endocytoscope with 450x magnification on a 14-inch monitor. The observation area of the epithelial surface is 400 $\times$ 400 μm^2. The outer diameter of the scope is 11.6 mm, and it has a 2.8-mm working channel. The video processor allows narrow-band imaging. The images are displayed on the monitor at a rate of 30 frames per second, the same frame rate as in routine video endoscopy. The two endoscopy systems were mounted in a single forward-viewing endoscope, and observation can be done either with a regular magnifying endoscopy system or with an endocytoscope. Inoue and colleagues[17] reported in vivo observation of the esophageal lesions with this integrated endocytoscope. About 28 patients with specific esophageal lesions that were detected by chromoendoscopy or narrow-band imaging, or both, were further evaluated by using endocytoscopy, followed by tissue biopsy or resection. The reported overall accuracy of endocytoscopy in differentiating between nonmalignant and malignant pathology was 82%, with the mean examination time of 9 minutes for a complete upper-gastrointestinal endoscopy. The author proposed a classification of the endocytoscopic images of atypia into five grades based on the shape and size of the cells and nuclei. Eberl and colleagues[18] confirmed those data by conducting a prospective study. An endoscopist who is aware of the endocytoscopic image analyzed 25 patients with esophageal lesions, and biopsy specimens were taken within the suspicious lesions. The diagnosis derived from the endocytoscopic images were compared with histologic findings as the gold standard. The sensitivity and specificity for the evaluation of the blinded pathologist was 81%, and 100%, respectively in the esophagus. If an endoscopist evaluated the endocytoscopic images in combination with the macroscopic endoscopic images, the sensitivity and specificity increased significantly. Pohl and colleagues[19] assessed the accuracy of endocytoscopy in correlation with histology in patients with Barrett's esophagus. Endocytoscopic images were recorded from areas in Barrett's segment without visible lesions, and biopsies were taken from the same area for precise comparison with histology. About 166 biopsy sites from 16 patients were analyzed. Adenocarcinoma was histologically diagnosed in 4.2% of biopsy sites, high-grade intraepithelial neoplasia, in 16.9%, and low-grade intraepithelial neoplasia, in 12.1%. Adequate assessment of endocytoscopic images was impossible in 49% of the area with magnification x450 and in 22% with magnification x1125. Only 23% of the images with lower magnification were interpretable to identify characteristics of neoplasia, and 41%, with higher magnification. Interobserver agreement was fair. Positive and negative predictive values for high-grade intraepithelial neoplasia or cancer were 0.29 and 0.83, respectively, for magnification x450 and 0.44 and 0.83, respectively, for magnification x1125. The investigators concluded that when not supported by macroscopic evidence, endoscopic histology using endocytoscopy lacks sufficient image quality to be of use in identifying neoplastic areas. This study is the first systematic evaluation of endocytoscopy in terms of applying it for surveillance purpose in which macroscopically normal mucosa were assessed. Pohl's study indicated that endocytoscopy is still not ready as a general surveillance tool, and it seems important to improve the accurate detection rate of the malignant lesions with low magnification within Barrett's segment. Endocytoscopy enables the direct visualization of living cells during endoscopy; however, only a limited area could be visualized each time. It may be more useful when we use this modality for a target inspection of the lesion after primary detection using other techniques such as narrow-band imaging or autofluorescence imaging, which provide a wider overview. There are other challenges lying ahead before endocytoscopy becomes clinically applicable, which are image stabilization, standardization of terminology, reproducibility of classification systems, and required use of methylene blue stain, which can potentially cause DNA damage in the tissue.[20] Another potential limitation would be the inability to visualize beyond the superficial layer of the epithelium. Image quality will be problematic especially during in vivo observation, because motility and cardiac impulses make it difficult to maintain adequate contact of the surface and to obtain interpretable clear images. In our current experience, we have succeeded in obtaining clear interpretable still images from endoscopically resected specimens of the Barrett's esophagus (**Figs. 3** and **4**). Our experiences imply that the problem of imaging quality during observation is not associated with the modality itself, because good-quality still images were taken even from small endoscopically resected specimen. We could see the architectural

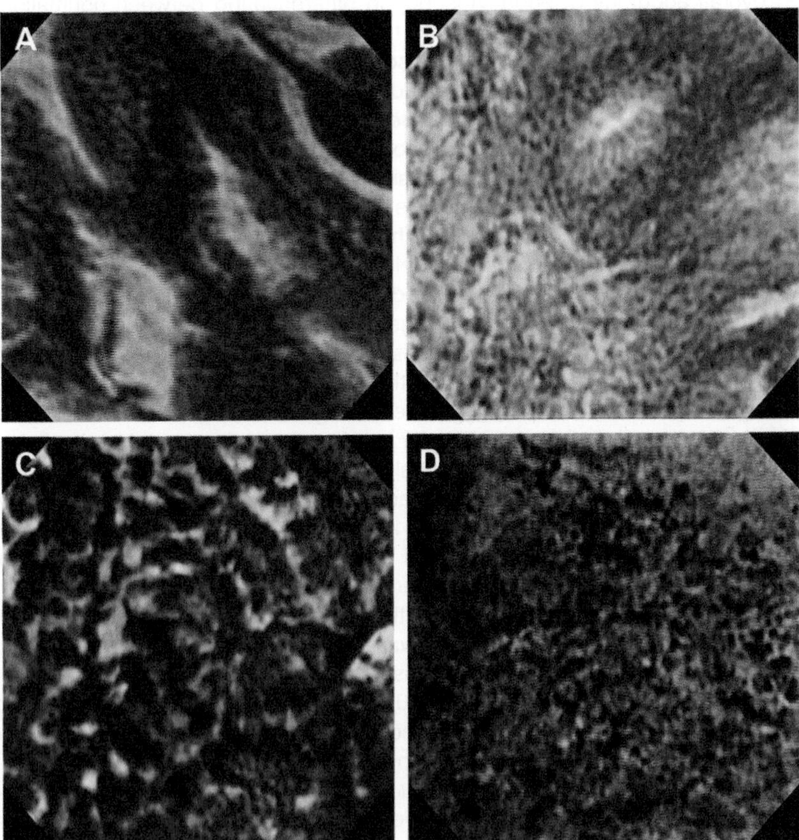

Fig. 3. Classification of endocytoscopic images of Barrett's esophagus with magnification x 450. (*A*). Barrett's esophagus without dysplasia: Gland appearance with uniform architecture. (*B*). Barrett's esophagus with low-grade dysplasia: Crowd gland appearance with maintained architecture; mild increased cellularity. (*C*). Barrett's esophagus with high-grade dysplasia: Crowd gland appearance with disordered architecture; moderate increased cellularity. (*D*). Esophageal adenocarcinoma: Total loss of gland appearance and architecture; severe increased cellularity.

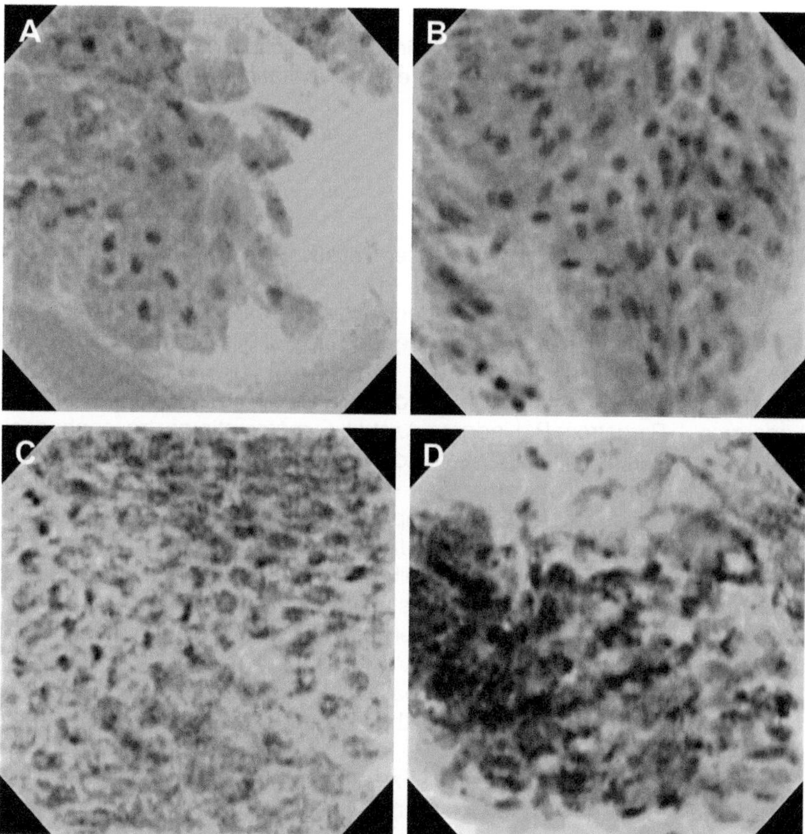

Fig. 4. Classification of endocytoscopic images of Barrett's esophagus with magnification x 1125. (*A*). Barrett's esophagus without dysplasia: Normal nucleus (N)/cytoplasm (*C*) ratio (hallo appearance). (*B*). Barrett's esophagus with low-grade dysplasia: Mild increased N/C ratio and mild disordered polarity; mitotic division appearance may be seen. (*C*). Barrett's esophagus with high-grade dysplasia: Moderately increased N/C ratio and moderate disordered polarity; mitotic division appearances are more prominent. (*D*). Esophageal adenocarcinoma: Severe increased N/C ratio and total loss of polarity.

characteristics of Barrett's mucosa between their stages with magnification x 450 and different characteristics of the cellular level with magnification x 1125. In other words, low magnification provides a more histologic insight into the tissue compared with high magnification, which shows more cytologic clues. We also faced difficulties in distinguishing between low-grade dysplasia and high-grade dysplasia, and between high-grade dysplasia and adenocarcinoma, especially with low magnification It will be essential to establish a usable classification technique before this technique can be implemented in practice. Cellular-level observation with endoscopy is an important step, and being able to acquire a "virtual histology" could greatly advance the care of patients with mucosal neoplastic disease.

SUMMARY

Endocytoscopy has been applied to detect lesions in the esophagus. It enables a real-time microscopic observation of living cells and has the potential to assess histological changes. Although there have been several promising data, challenges still lie before endocytoscopy becomes clinically applicable. Image stabilization and reproducibility of classification systems are major limitations. Further research effort toward these challenges is needed.

REFERENCES

1. Jamel A, Siegel R, Wald E, et al. Cancer statistics. CA Cancer J Clin 2008;58(2): 71–96.
2. Brown L, Devesa S, Chow WH. Incidence of adenocarcinoma of the esophagus among white Americans by sex, stage, and age. J Natl Cancer Inst 2008;100: 1184–7.
3. Enzinger P, Mayer R. Esophageal cancer. N Engl J Med 2003;349:2241–52.
4. Lagergren J, Bergstrom R, Lindgren A, et al. Symptomatic gastroesophageal reflux as a risk factor for esophageal adenocarcinoma. N Engl J Med 1999;340: 825–31.
5. Shaheen N, Ransohoff D. Gastroesophageal reflux, Barrett's esophagus and esophageal cancer, scientific review. JAMA 2002;287:1972–81.
6. Mashimo H, Wagh M, Goyal R. Surveillance and screening for Barrett's esophagus and adenocarcinoma. J Clin Gastroenterol 2005;39:S33–41.
7. Wang K, Sampliner R. Updated guidelines 2008 for the diagnosis, surveillance and therapy of Barrett's esophagus. Am J Gastroenterol 2008;103:788–97.
8. Eloubeidi M, Provenzale D. Does this patient have Barrett's esophagus? The utility of predicting Barrett's esophagus at the index endoscopy. Am J Gastroenterol 1999;94:937–43.
9. Buttar N, Wang K, Burgart L, et al. Extent of high grade dysplasia in Barrett's esophagus correlated with risk of adenocarcinoma. Gastroenterology 2001;120: 1630–9.
10. Curvers W, Kiesslich R, Bergman J. Novel imaging modalities in the detection of oesophageal neoplasia. Best Pract Res Clin Gastroenterol 2008;22:687–720.
11. Andrea M, Dias O, Santos A. A contact endoscopy of the vocal cord: normal and pathological patterns. Acta Otolaryngol 1995;115:314–6.
12. Andrea M, Dias O, Santos A. A contact endoscopy during microlaryngeal surgery: a new technique for endoscopic examination of the larynx. Ann Otol Rhinol Laryngol 1995;104:333–9.
13. Inoue H, Kudo SE, Shiokawa A. Technology insight: laser-scanning confocal microscopy and endocytoscopy for cellular observation of the gastrointestinal tract. Nat Clin Pract Gastroenterol Hepatol 2005;2:31–7.
14. Inoue H, Kudo SE, Shiokawa A. Novel endoscopic imaging techniques toward in vivo observation of living cancer cells in the gastrointestinal tract. Clin Gastroenterol Helpatol 2005;3:S61–3.
15. Kumagai Y, Monma K, Kawada K. Magnifying chromoendoscopy of the esophagus: in-vivo pathological diagnosis using an endocytoscopy system. Endoscopy 2004;36:590–4.
16. Inoue H, Kazawa T, Sato Y, et al. In vivo observation of living cancer cells in the esophagus, stomach, and colon using catheter-type contact endoscope, "endocytoscopy system". Gastrointest Endosc Clin N Am 2004;14:589–94.
17. Inoue H, Sasajima K, Kaga M, et al. Endoscopic in vivo evaluation of tissue atypia in the esophagus using a newly designed integrated endocytoscope: a pilot trial. Endoscopy 2006;38:891–5.

18. Eberl T, Jechart G, Probst A, et al. Can an endocytoscope system (ECS) predict histology in neoplastic lesions? Endoscopy 2007;39:497–501.
19. Pohl H, Koch M, Khalifa A, et al. Evaluation of endocytoscopy in the surveillance of patients with Barrett's esophagus. Endoscopy 2007;39:492–6.
20. Olliver J, Wild C, Sahay P, et al. Chromoendoscopy with methylene blue and associated DNA damage in Barrett's esophagus. Lancet 2003;362:373–4.

Targeted Endoscopic Imaging

Meng Li, PhD[a], Thomas D. Wang, MD, PhD[b,c,*]

KEYWORDS

• Endoscopy • Molecular imaging • Targets • Early detection

Endoscopic detection of disease in the digestive tract is currently being performed using visualization and interpretation of white light images reflected from the mucosal surface in real time.[1] In the esophagus, tissue transforms from normal to malignant by passing through a sequence of histologic stages that include squamous, metaplasia, dysplasia, and carcinoma[2] (**Fig. 1**). The physician makes diagnostic decisions and determines the site for biopsy based on architectural appearance, including mass effect, texture variations, and color changes. This strategy has resulted in widespread use of endoscopy to perform surveillance, stage disease, and apply therapy; the diagnostic information provided by this approach comes primarily from structural changes in the tissue, such as size, shape, and number. In the absence of these changes, biopsies may be performed in a random fashion, such as in the setting of Barrett's esophagus and ulcerative colitis, whereby effectiveness is significantly limited by sampling error.[3,4] Unfortunately, this strategy alone does not take advantage of the significant wealth of undiscovered information contained within the molecular properties of tissue that can reveal details about mucosal function, if properly imaged. Over the past few decades, we have gained a tremendous amount of knowledge about the molecular processes involved in cancer biology. It is now known that cancer results from a number and variety of molecular and cellular changes that arise from a gradual accumulation of genetic changes.[5] Thus, the ability to acquire real time data about the molecular expression of cells and tissues within the digestive tract can allow physicians to improve patient management strategies. For example, observing the molecular expression pattern of premalignant (dysplastic) mucosa can provide new methods

This work was supported by grant nos. K08 DK067618 and R03 CA096752 from the National Institutes of Health and the Clinical Scientist Translational Research Award from Doris Duke Charitable Foundation.

[a] Division of Gastroenterology and Hepatology, Department of Medicine, University of Michigan School of Medicine, 109 Zina Pitcher Place, BSRB 1722, Ann Arbor, MI 48109, USA

[b] Division of Gastroenterology and Hepatology, Department of Medicine, University of Michigan School of Medicine, 109 Zina Pitcher Place, BSRB 1522, Ann Arbor, MI 48109, USA

[c] Department of Biomedical Engineering, University of Michigan, 109 Zina Pitcher Place, Ann Arbor, MI 48109, USA

* Corresponding author. Division of Gastroenterology and Hepatology, University of Michigan School of Medicine, 109 Zina Pitcher Place, BSRB 1522, Ann Arbor, MI 48109.

E-mail address: thomaswa@umich.edu (T.D. Wang).

Gastrointest Endoscopy Clin N Am 19 (2009) 283–298

doi:10.1016/j.giec.2009.02.001

giendo.theclinics.com

1052-5157/09/$ – see front matter

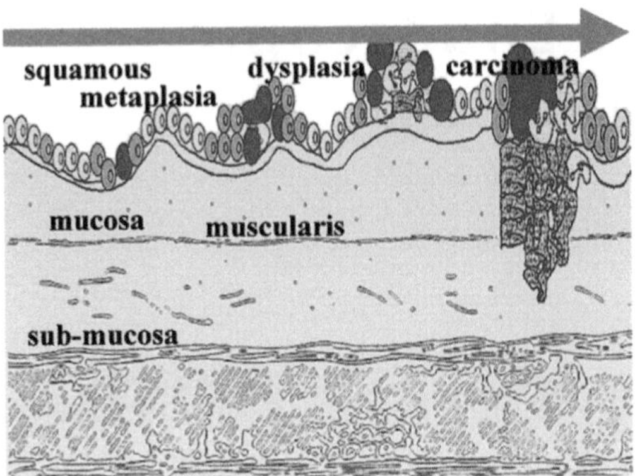

Fig. 1. Cancer transformation in the digestive tract. Progression from normal to malignant mucosa in the esophagus passes through histologic stages of squamous, metaplasia, dysplasia, and carcinoma. Molecular variations occur well in advance of morphologic changes, providing a window of opportunity to perform earlier detection and therapy.

for the early detection of cancer, and interval imaging of expressed targets can allow physicians to monitor the efficacy of therapy. In essence, changes in molecular expression occur well before that of structural features, thus greater knowledge at an earlier time may be the key to changing the course of disease progression.

Molecular changes in diseased cells within the mucosa can be present either inside the cell or on its surface. A significant advantage for performing targeted imaging in the mucosa of the digestive tract is the opportunity to apply exogenous probes topically. This method of administration can focus the investigation on a specific region of involvement, is much less likely to develop an immunogenic reaction, and can more easily overcome regulatory hurdles. The best studied intracellular targets are proteolytic enzymes and the most established cell surface targets are transmembrane proteins and glycoproteins. These structures are too small to be visualized directly, even with the highest resolution imaging instruments. Instead, exogenous probes labeled with fluorescent dyes that interact with these targets are needed to detect their presence. Several different classes of probe technologies have been evaluated for performing targeted imaging, in small animals and human subjects. For example, monoclonal antibodies have been investigated for tumor detection and drug delivery because of their high specificity.[6,7] However, their use in vivo has been limited by delivery challenges, immunogenicity, and cost for reagent development. Recently, several near-infrared fluorescent imaging probes directed toward intracellular targets have been developed to detect neoplasia on fluorescence endoscopy.[8] These molecular targets include proteolytic enzymes,[9] matrix metalloproteinases,[10] endothelial-specific markers,[11] and apoptosis reporters.[12,13]

MOLECULAR TARGETS

Molecular targets provide useful information about the tissue phenotype and are overexpressed in transformed mucosa relative to normal. There has been great progress in unraveling the sequence of genetic changes that lead to clonal selection and growth advantages for cells in the mucosa of the digestive tract that transform into cancer.[14,15] Moreover, there is now a greater understanding of the timing of molecular changes that occur early, such as alterations in p53 and p16, versus late, such as loss of heterozygosity and cell cycle checkpoints.[16,17] This ability to acquire this information on imaging has significant implications on risk stratifying patients who have a higher likelihood for developing cancer, such as those with Barrett's esophagus, atrophic gastritis, and ulcerative colitis. Initial efforts in developing this novel, targeted, endoscopic imaging strategy have focused on several overexpressed intracellular and cell surface receptors. These targets include cathepsin B,[18,19] matrix metalloproteinases (MMPs),[20,21] carcinoembryonic antigen (CEA),[22,23] MUC1 and MUC2,[24,25] and HER2/neu (ERBB2),[26,27] and they play a significant role in cancer transformation of mucosa in the digestive tract.

Proteases

Proteases are proteolytic enzymes that play an important role in cell proliferation, invasion, apoptosis, angiogenesis, and metastasis, and they form important targets for the detection and diagnosis of cancer in the digestive tract. In particular, they have been shown to be overexpressed in the development of colon cancer. For example, cathepsin B has been shown to be up-regulated in areas of inflammation, necrosis, angiogenesis, dysplasia, and carcinoma. In addition, metalloproteinases are believed to be targets of the Wnt signaling pathway.[28] The ability of protease-sensitive probes to improve detection of adenomas, in which cathepsin B is overexpressed, has been demonstrated in the small bowel of $Apc^{Min/+}$ mice.[29] In this ex vivo study, the smallest lesion detectable was found to be 50 μm in diameter. Furthermore, the use of protease-sensitive probes to detect colonic neoplasia in vivo on wide-area endoscopy has been shown using colonic tumor cells implanted into the small bowel of an animal model.[30] This combination of white light reflectance and near-infrared fluorescence images of colonic mucosa demonstrates the integration of structural and functional data using protease-activated interactions to illustrate this imaging strategy. This study showed that increased near-infrared fluorescence intensity could be used to detect overexpression of cathepsin B and its related activity in neoplastic compared with normal mucosa.

Antibody Targets

The first attempts to detect cell surface targets that are overexpressed in neoplastic compared with normal mucosa used monoclonal antibodies as affinity probes. Most of these targets are membrane-associated glycoproteins, and the synthesis and secretion of these high-molecular weight biomolecules are common features of all glandular epithelial tissues. CEA is a glycoprotein that is involved in cell adhesion, and is found to be increased in the serum of individuals with colorectal, gastric, pancreatic, lung, and breast carcinomas.[31] The serum level of CEA typically normalizes after tumor resection, thus any subsequent elevation suggests cancer recurrence. CEA levels may also be increased in some nonneoplastic conditions, such as ulcerative colitis, pancreatitis, and cirrhosis. Mucins, such as MUC1, are also membrane glycoproteins commonly found on epithelial cells and are anchored to the apical surface by a transmembrane domain.[24] This protein provides a protective function to the cells by binding to pathogens and also performs cell signaling. Overexpression, aberrant intracellular localization, and changes in glycosylation of this protein have been associated with adenocarcinoma. MUC2 produces a secreted mucin protein that forms an insoluble mucous barrier to protect the gut lumen.[25] In patients with gastric cancer, the expression of MUC1 is associated with invasive proliferation and a poor outcome, whereas expression of MUC2 is related to noninvasive growth and a favorable prognosis. Colorectal carcinomas show a high level of expression of fully glycosylated MUC1 in advanced stages or in metastatic lesions. In addition, the expression of sialylated MUC1 mucin is strongly correlated with poor outcome in patients with intrahepatic bile duct carcinoma.

Peptide Targets

HER2/neu (ERBB2) is a plasma membrane receptor in the epidermal growth factor family that is normally associated with cell signaling involving the mitogen-activated protein kinase (MAPK) pathway and is also believed to activate PI3 K/Akt signaling.[26] This protooncogene plays an important role in promoting neoplastic progression in the esophagus by gene amplification and is associated with inhibition of apoptosis and enhanced cell proliferation.[32,33] HER-2/neu signaling increases MMP activity, enhances tumorigenic and metastatic potential, and is a potent inducer of VEGF and tumor vascularity.[34] Gene amplification of HER2/neu is a common mechanism for the development of esophageal adenocarcinoma, and the associated gene is found to be amplified in 15% to 25% of esophageal cancers.[35] HER2/neu is also amplified in approximately 25% to 30% of human breast cancers, and results in the overexpression of the associated receptor, which is a well-established target for trastuzumab (Herceptin), a humanized monoclonal antibody.[36] In addition, small molecules, such as lapatinib, are being developed as a novel therapy for inhibiting tyrosine kinase activity by blocking the ATP-binding site.[37] Clinical studies for treating patients with esophageal adenocarcinoma who are HER2/neu positive with trastuzumab and lapatinib are underway.

MOLECULAR PROBES

Intracellular and cell surface targets are typically too small in size to be visualized directly, and require the use of exogenous probes that become optically active after interacting with specific biomolecules that are overexpressed in neoplastic compared with normal tissues. Probe characteristics that are promising for use in the digestive tract include (1) high diversity, (2) affinity binding, (3) rapid kinetics (time scale of minutes), (4) deep tissue penetration, (5) low immunogenicity, (6) capacity for large scale synthesis, (7) easy to label, and (8) low cost. The choice of the fluorescence label depends on the type of molecular interactions to be measured, and the wavelength of the instrument being used for excitation and emission. Visible agents, such as fluorescein derivatives, provide the best image resolution and are easy to conjugate, whereas near-infrared probes provide the deepest tissue penetration and least autofluorescence background.

Proteases

Proteases are intracellular targets whose enzymatic activity creates a biochemical interaction that stimulates the molecular probe to emit light. These probes have been designed to produce near-infrared fluorescence after proteolytic cleavage, and exist in several forms, including auto-quenched, self-quenched, dual-labeled, and cell-penetrating.[38] One of the advantages of activatable probes is that a single enzyme can cleave multiple fluorophores to provide signal amplification and achieve high target-to-background ratios. This property of activatable probes results in the use of lower doses than with nonactivatable imaging probes, such as antibodies and peptides. A robust signal is critical for observing intracellular processes because the target concentration in this environment is typically low. Additional probe properties that require consideration include clearance, binding kinetics, degradation susceptibility, and extent of nonspecific accumulation. Prosense (VisEn Medical, Inc, Bedford, Massachusetts) is an intravenously injected, activatable probe that consists of a synthetic graft poly-L-lysine copolymer that is sterically protected by multiple methoxypolyethylene glycol side chains and has multiple near-infrared fluorochromes.[39] A variety of proteases, in particular cathepsin B, can cleave the lysine-lysine bonds, and amplify the fluorescence signal by a factor of 15 to 30. Prosense 680 and 750 have a maximum absorption at 680 and 750 nm, respectively, and a peak emission at 700 and 780 nm, respectively. The performance of these probes has been demonstrated endoscopically in genetically engineered mice.

Antibody Targets

Antibody probes are gamma globulins that affinity bind to antigenic targets expressed on the cell surface. Light chains are basic structural units of the antibody whose tips express a wide variety of amino acid sequences that can form highly specific ionic and covalent bonds with the molecular targets. The number of different combinations of amino acid sequences defines the variability (diversity), and allows for antibodies to bind to a large number of different targets. A monoclonal mouse anti-CEA antibody has been developed to perform targeted endoscopic imaging of colonic neoplasia. The fluorescence label consists of 5(6)-carboxyfluorescein-*N*-hydroxysuccinimide ester (FLUOS), and has maximum excitation and emission wavelengths of 494 and 518 nm, respectively.[40] The anti-CEA antibody was labeled with FLUOS using a 1:10 molar reaction for a period of 2 hours, and was then purified by gel filtration on a Sephadex column to achieve a final concentration of approximately 1 mg/mL. The probe was also mixed with mucilago tylose, a gel containing methylhydroxyethylcellulose and carboxymethylcellulose in a 4% solution to increase the viscosity of the solution before in vivo application. In addition, quinoline yellow was added to this mixture to form a 1% solution.

Antibodies have also been labeled with indocyanine green (ICG) derivatives for targeting the detection of cancer in the digestive tract. ICG is a near-infrared dye that has a maximum absorption at 805 nm and a peak emission at 835 nm. It has been approved by the US Food and Drug Administration (FDA) for intravenous use to measure cardiac output, assess hepatic function, and visualize ocular vessels. ICG derivatives including ICG-*N*-hydroxysulfosuccinimide ester (ICG-sulfo-OSu) and 3-ICG-acyl-1,3-thiazolidine-2-thione (ICG-ATT) have been developed for labeling monoclonal antibodies.[41] Antibody probes that have been developed in this manner include anti-CEA and anti-MUC1. These compounds incur small shifts in the excitation and emission wavelengths relative to pure ICG, and have been used to demonstrate proof of principle for targeted endoscopic imaging.

Peptide Targets

Peptides have several advantages for performing targeted detection in the digestive tract because of their high diversity, rapid binding kinetics, and potential for deep diffusion in diseased mucosa.[42] In addition, peptides can be labeled easily and are generally nontoxic and nonimmunogenic. Peptides have been selected using techniques of phage display, a powerful combinatorial method that uses recombinant DNA technology to generate a library of clones that bind preferentially to the cell surface. The protein coat of bacteriophage, such as the filamentous M13 oricosahedral T7, is genetically engineered to express a high diversity ($>10^9$) of unique peptide sequences. Selection of peptides that affinity bind to overexpressed cell surface targets is then performed by biopanning the library against normal and diseased cells and tissues. The DNA sequences are then recovered and used to synthesize the candidate peptides with the addition of a fluorescent label. Techniques of phage display have been successfully used to identify peptides that bind preferentially to dysplastic rather than to normal mucosa in the colon and esophagus. The peptides with the highest target-to-background ratio relative to control cells are selected for clinical use. Using this selection strategy for dysplastic esophageal mucosa, the phage with the peptide sequence ASYNYDA was identified and found using a Basic Local Alignment Search Tool (BLAST) search to have binding homology with protocadherin gamma.[43] Similarly, the peptide with sequence VRPMPLQ was selected for affinity binding to dysplastic colonic mucosa, and was found on BLAST to have binding homology with the laminin-G domain of contactin-associated protein (Caspr-1).[44]

MOLECULAR IMAGING INSTRUMENTS

Wide-Area Endoscopy

Wide-area endoscopy provides high-resolution images on the macroscopic scale (millimeters to centimeters) to rapidly survey large surface areas of mucosa in the digestive tract to localize regions suspicious for disease. The instrument design will depend on the fluorescence excitation and emission wavelengths of the labeled probe, and involves a trade-off between image resolution and autofluorescence background. Visible probes, such as fluorescein derivatives, require excitation and provide emission at approximately 488 nm and 510 nm, respectively. This regime provides the best image resolution but generates the most autofluorescence background. Near-infrared probes, such as ICG derivatives, provide less image resolution but generate virtually no autofluorescence background.

Proteases

For imaging of proteases using activatable probes, techniques of wide-area endoscopy have been developed to collect near-infrared fluorescence images in small animal models. This microcatheter instrument consists of 10,000 collection fibers surrounded by 14 illumination fibers and is contained within a 0.8-mm diameter sheath with a working length of 100 cm.[30] The tip of the catheter is fused to an objective lens that is 0.4 mm in diameter and has a 0.35-mm focal length. Fluorescence excitation is provided by a mercury vapor lamp by way of a 670-nm short pass filter. The light is first collimated with an aspheric lens, and delivered through a 5-mm diameter, liquid light guide with numeric aperture of 0.55. The light collected by the image guide is separated by a 670-nm dichroic mirror into a white light component between 400 and 650 nm and fluorescence emission at wavelengths longer than 670 nm, which is then band-pass filtered between 690 and 800 nm. Two separate collecting lens systems then relay the white light and fluorescence images onto a standard video camera and a near-infrared fluorescence camera, respectively.

Antibody targets

The endoscopic instrument for imaging cell surface targets with monoclonal antibodies uses visible fluorescence excitation that is provided by a halogen source whereby the light passes through a 490-nm narrow band filter.[40] The emission from the fluorescence labeled anti-CEA antibody is collected by a conventional fiber-optic endoscope. This fluorescence light passes through a 520-nm narrow band filter, and the images are captured by a single reflex 35-mm camera attached to the proximal end of the endoscope. Conventional white light endoscopy is performed first, and the illumination is turned off when the fluorescein-labeled anti-CEA antibody is topically applied to the mucosal surface for an incubation time of approximately 10 minutes followed by rinsing of the unbound antibodies with 0.9% saline solution.

For imaging with near-infrared fluorescence-labeled antibodies, a prototype endoscope has been developed that uses a 300-W xenon lamp as a light source.[45] The excitation band is determined by a 710- to 790-nm barrier filter placed between the lamp and the endoscope. There is an additional filter in front of the lamp to block infrared light from reaching the white light camera. Fluorescence is collected in the 810- to 920-nm band with a barrier filter placed in front of an intensified charge-coupled device (CCD) camera. This detection unit, along with the white light camera, is attached to the proximal end of the endoscope with an adapter. The captured white light and fluorescence images are relayed by way of a control unit to an image capturing device and magneto-optical disk drive subsystem for recording and storing the images.

Peptide targets

For imaging of peptide targets, a prototype wide-area endoscope has been developed that collects fluorescence from peptides labeled with fluorescein derivatives. This instrument can image in three different modes, including white light (WL), narrow-band imaging (NBI), and fluorescence imaging.[46] In the WL mode, the full visible spectrum from 400 to 700 nm is collected, whereas in the NBI mode, a set of spectral bands in the red, green, and blue regimes is detected. In the fluorescence mode, a filter wheel enters the illumination path, and provides fluorescence excitation in the 395- to 475-nm band. In addition, illumination from 525 to 575 nm provides reflected light in the green spectral regime centered at 550 nm. The fluorescence image is collected by the peripherally located CCD detector, which has a 490- to 625-nm band-pass filter for blocking the excitation light. Normal mucosa emits bright autofluorescence, thus the composite color appears as bright green. Because the increased vasculature in neoplastic mucosa absorbs autofluorescence, it appears with decreased intensity. The WL and NBI images are collected by the center objective lens, and the fluorescence image is collected by a second objective lens located near the periphery. A xenon light source provides the illumination for all three modes, which are determined by the filter wheel located in the image processor. Illumination for all three modes of imaging is delivered through the two fiber-optic light guides. Furthermore, there is a 2.8-mm diameter instrument channel, which can be used to deliver either a confocal microendoscope or biopsy forceps. The objectives are forward viewing and have a field of view (FOV), defined by a maximum angle of illumination of 140°.

Confocal Microscopy

Confocal microscopy uses the core of an optical fiber as a pinhole, placed between the objective lens and the detector, to allow only the light that originates from within a tiny volume below the mucosal surface to be collected.[47] All other sources of scattered light do not have the correct path to be detected, and thus become spatially filtered. This process creates a high-resolution image from a thin section within otherwise optically thick tissue, and is known as optical sectioning. Because of the subcellular resolution that can be achieved with this technique, it is particularly useful for validating probe binding to cells in the mucosa rather than accumulating nonspecifically in mucus and debris. Moreover, the images can be collected at sufficiently fast frame rates to observe biologic behavior with minimal disturbance from motion artifacts caused by peristalsis using high-speed scanning mechanisms. Recent advancements in miniaturization of optics, the availability of fiber optics, and the emergence of microscanners have allowed the technique of confocal microscopy to be performed in vivo through medical endoscopes to perform rapid, real-time optical assessment of tissue pathology.[48] This approach represents a significant advance in endoscopic screening for the early detection of cancer by providing a new method that can increase the yield of physical biopsy, reduce the risks of screening (ie, bleeding, infection, and perforation), and lower the cost of processing tissue pathology.

The Cellvizio (Mauna Kea Technologies, Paris, France) is an endoscope-compatible confocal microscope; it has an imaging bundle with ~30,000 optical fibers and uses a gradient index (GRIN) microlens to focus the beam.[49] There are two versions of the miniprobe, called S and HD: the S version has a working distance of 0 μm, transverse resolution of 5 μm, and axial resolution of 15 μm; the HD version has a working distance of 50 μm, transverse resolution of 2.5 μm, and axial resolution of 20 μm. Images are collected in a horizontal plane (en face) at 12 frames per second with a field of view of either 600 × 500 or 240 × 200 μm^2. Fluorescence is collected by the same optical fibers and transmitted back to the detector. A long-pass filter rejects the excitation light, and fluorescence is detected with an avalanche photodiode. The image processing performed includes subtraction of fiber autofluorescence and calibration of individual fiber transmission efficiencies. The fibered confocal miniprobe has the size and flexibility to pass through the instrument channel, and can be accurately placed onto the mucosa using guidance from the white light image. The frame rate is adequate to achieve consistent images with little interference from motion artifacts.

IN VIVO MOLECULAR IMAGING

Proteases

In vivo imaging of protease activity has been demonstrated in an orthotopic colon cancer model. The mucosa of the descending colon in C57BL6/J mice was injected with 1 × 10^6 CT26 murine colon cancer cells by way of a midline incision.[30] After 13 days to allow for tumor growth, Prosense 680, a protease-activated probe sensitive to cathepsin B, was injected intravenously at a concentration of 2 nmol in a volume of 150 μL, and small-animal endoscopy was performed the next day. An increase in near-infrared fluorescence was detected at the site of the tumor, as shown in **Fig. 2**. **Fig 2**A and D show the in vivo white light endoscopic images of normal and cancerous murine colonic mucosa, respectively. **Fig. 2**B shows no fluorescence from normal mucosa, whereas **Fig. 2**E reveals a region of increased near-infrared fluorescence provided by cathepsin B activity at the site of the tumor. **Fig. 2**F shows a false color overlay of white light and fluorescence images to register the site of the tumor with that of the fluorescence. Combining the white light and fluorescence images integrates anatomic features from structural changes in the mucosa with functional data provided by protease activity, allowing for identification of smaller, flat lesions, which may not be detected on white light endoscopy alone.

Antibody Targets

The use of topically applied fluorescence-labeled anti-CEA antibody to target the detection of dysplasia on wide-area endoscopy has been demonstrated in vivo in the colon.[40] If a lesion was found on white light endoscopy, approximately 2 to 6 mL of the fluorescein-labeled anti-CEA antibody mixed with mucilago tylose was topically applied to the surrounding mucosa. An increased fluorescence signal was detected in 19 of the 25 carcinomas and in three of eight adenomas. A white light endoscopic image of a colonic adenoma is shown in **Fig. 3**A, and reveals the presence of a mass lesion. The corresponding fluorescence image collected after topical incubation with the labeled anti-CEA antibody shown in **Fig. 3**B reveals increased intensity at the site of the lesion. Only one out of six adenocarcinomas that did not reveal increased fluorescence showed overexpression of CEA on immunohistochemistry. The other fluorescence-negative carcinomas showed either ulceration or spontaneous bleeding without CEA reactivity in areas of tumor on immunohistochemistry. Four of the fluorescence-negative adenomas were classified histologically as low-grade

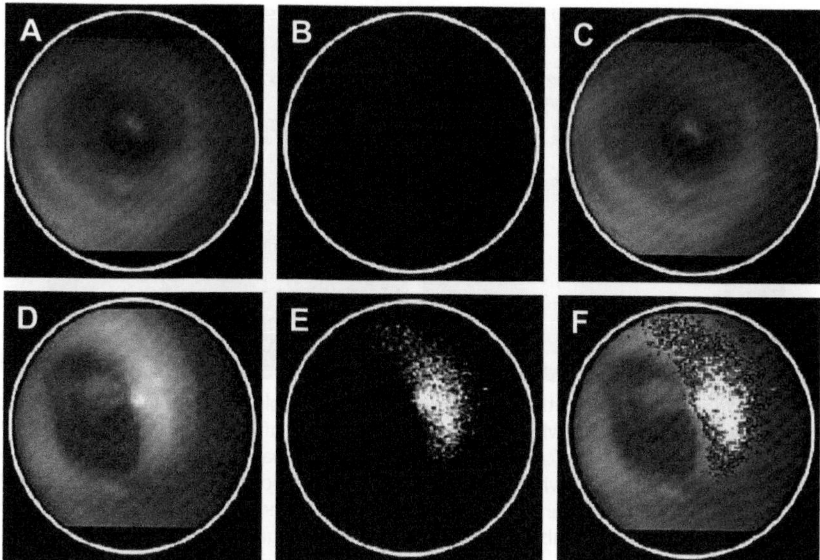

Fig. 2. Near-infrared endoscopic imaging of protease activity in a small animal model. Increase in near-infrared fluorescence intensity reveals protease activity from a colonic adenocarcinoma (*bottom row*) in comparison to normal colonic mucosa (*top row*) in an orthotopically implanted mouse model. (*A, D*) In vivo white light endoscopic images of normal (*A*) and cancerous (*D*) murine colonic mucosa. (*B, E*) Near-infrared fluorescence images following intravenous injection of Prosense 680, a protease activated probe sensitive to cathepsin B, showing increased intensity at the site of the tumor but not in normal mucosa. (*C, F*) False color overlay of white light with fluorescence images showing integration of structural and functional data. (*From* Alencar H, Funovics MA, Figueiredo J, et al. Colonic adenocarcinomas: near-infrared microcatheter imaging of smart probes for early detection—study in mice. Radiology 2007;244(1):236; with permission.)

dysplasia. The normal-appearing colonic mucosa immediately surrounding the 33 colorectal lesions did not show any significantly increased fluorescence intensity. The experimental portion of the study extended the duration of colonoscopy by approximately 15 to 30 minutes. An evaluation using the fluorescence endoscope was performed on the same specimens ex vivo immediately after resection and confirmed the in vivo results. Finally, the fluorescence intensity measured endoscopically had good correlation with CEA expression by the luminal epithelial cells on immunohistochemistry.

Monoclonal ICG-sulfo-OSu-labeled mouse anti-CEA antibody has also been used to target gastric cancer on biopsy specimens and imaged with near-infrared endoscopy.[41] Immunohistochemical analysis was first performed on the excised tissues to determine which gastric specimens overexpress CEA. These specimens positive for CEA were rinsed with warm water containing 2,000 U of pronase, 1 g of bicarbonate, and 4 mg of dimethylpolysiloxane for 15 minutes at room temperature. In addition, normal horse serum was administered to the specimens for 15 minutes to provide a nonspecific blocking agent. The mucosal surface was then incubated with monoclonal ICG-sulfo-OSu-labeled mouse anti-CEA antibody for 60 minutes. A conventional white light endoscopic image was collected first from freshly resected gastric mucosa, and then a near-infrared fluorescence image of the same specimen stained with ICG-sulfo-OSu-labeled anti-CEA antibody was acquired, revealing foci of cancer.

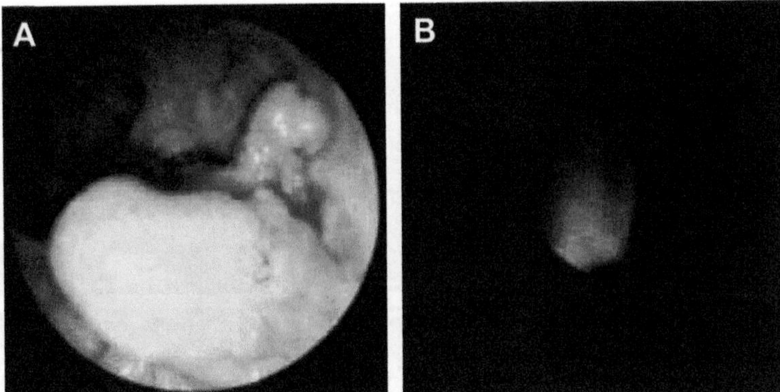

Fig. 3. In vivo localization of anti-CEA antibody binding to colonic adenoma on fluorescence endoscopy. (*A*) A conventional white light endoscopic image of a colonic adenoma reveals the presence of a mass lesion. (*B*) The corresponding fluorescence image collected in vivo after topical administration and incubation with the labeled anti-CEA antibody shows increased intensity at the site of the lesion. (*From* Keller R, Winde G, Terpe HJ, Foerster EC, Domschke W. Fluorescence endoscopy using a fluorescein-labeled monoclonal antibody against carcinoembryonic antigen in patients with colorectal carcinoma and adenoma. Endoscopy 2002;34(10):805; with permission.)

In addition, specimens of normal gastric mucosa did not reveal antibody binding, and were used as controls.

Peptide Targets

The use of topically applied fluorescence-labeled peptides to target the detection of high-grade dysplasia on wide-area endoscopy has been demonstrated in vivo in Barrett's esophagus.[43] With Institutional Review Board approval and informed consent, patients with a history of Barrett's esophagus and biopsy-proven high-grade dysplasia scheduled for endoscopic mucosal resection were recruited into the study. For each subject who enrolled in the study, complete blood count (CBC), platelets, and chemistries (Panel-7) were obtained, including blood urea nitrogen (BUN), creatinine (Cr), glucose (Glu), and liver function tests (LFTs), before and approximately 24 hours after the procedure to monitor for potential peptide toxicity. After esophageal intubation, a 10-second video was collected in white light mode. Then, approximately 3 mL of peptide with sequence ASYNYDA at a concentration of 10 μM was administered topically to the distal esophagus using a mist spray catheter. After 10 minutes for incubation, the unbound peptide was gently rinsed off with water, and another 10-second video of the fluorescence image was collected showing localized peptide binding. **Fig. 4**A shows a conventional white light image of Barrett's in the distal esophagus in vivo; no distinct architectural lesions can be seen. **Fig. 4**B shows the corresponding NBI image of the same region of the esophagus, and highlights the presence of intestinal metaplasia, as distinguished by the brown color, but this image is not sensitive to the presence of dysplasia. In **Fig. 4**C, the fluorescence image collected following topical administration and incubation of the peptide reveals a region of high-grade dysplasia. Targeted biopsies were then collected, and dysplasia was confirmed by two gastrointestinal pathologists.

The use of confocal microscopy to validate binding of topically applied fluorescence-labeled peptides to dysplastic crypts has been demonstrated in vivo with sporadic colonic adenomas.[44] After IRB approval and informed consent, adult

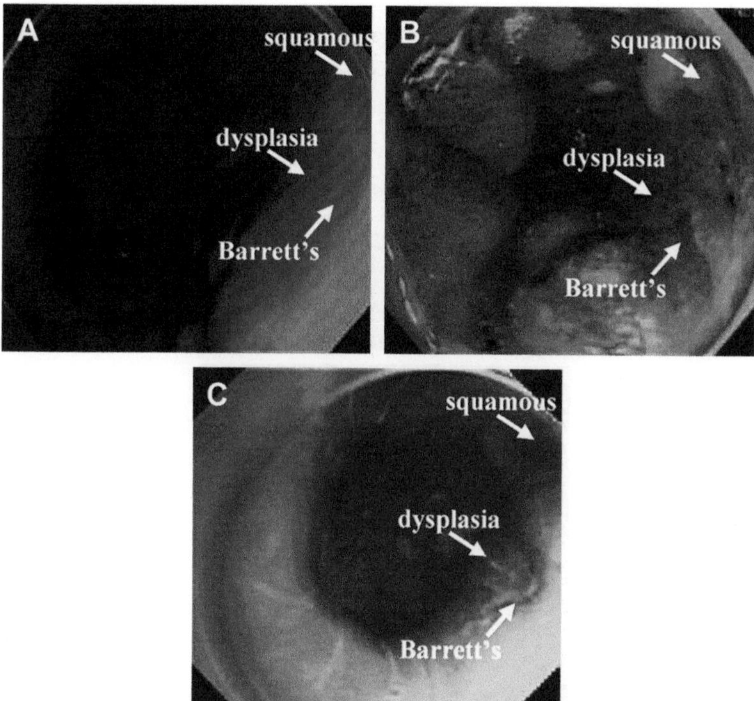

Fig. 4. In vivo localization of peptide binding to high-grade dysplasia in Barrett's esophagus on wide-area endoscopy. (*A*) A conventional white light endoscopic image of Barrett's esophagus shows no evidence of premalignant lesions. (*B*) NBI of the same region shows improved contrast, highlighting intestinal metaplasia but not dysplasia. (*C*) In vivo fluorescence image following topical administration and incubation with affinity peptide, sequence ASYNYDA, reveals foci of high-grade dysplasia.

patients already scheduled for screening colonoscopy were recruited into the study. The same blood tests described earlier were performed to monitor for peptide toxicity. If an adenoma was seen on white light colonoscopy, approximately 3 mL of the fluorescence-labeled peptide with sequence VRPMPLQ at a concentration of 100 μM was administered topically to the adenoma and surrounding normal mucosa. After 10 minutes for incubation, the unbound peptide was gently rinsed off with water, and the fibered confocal miniprobe was passed through the instrument channel, and placed into contact with the mucosa for collection of fluorescence images. **Fig. 5**A shows a white light endoscopic image of a colonic adenoma, used as a model for dysplasia. **Fig. 5**B shows an in vivo confocal image following staining with the fluorescence-labeled peptide; this image demonstrates binding to dysplastic crypts (left half) and no binding to normal (right half) crypts (scale bar 20 μm). **Fig. 5**C shows a confocal image with control peptide (scrambled) with sequence QLMRPPV and shows no binding.

REGULATORY OVERSIGHT

The knowledge to be gained by imaging the pattern of expression of molecular targets in the digestive tract is tremendous. However, caution must be exercised when pursuing investigation in human subjects to validate in vivo probe activity. The use

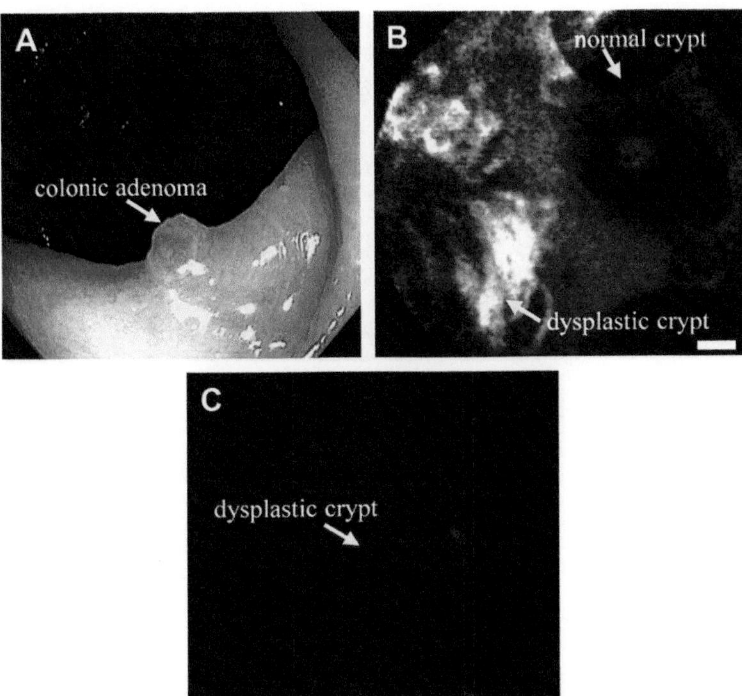

Fig. 5. In vivo validation of peptide binding to colonic adenoma on confocal microscopy. (*A*) Conventional white light endoscopic image of colonic adenoma. (*B*) In vivo confocal image following topical application and incubation of fluorescence-labeled affinity peptide, sequence VRPMPLQ, shows binding to dysplastic (*left half*) and no binding to normal (*right half*) crypts. (*C*) Confocal image with control peptide (scrambled), sequence QLMRPPV, shows no binding to adenoma (scale bar 20 μm). (*From* Hsiung PL, Hardy J, Friedland S, et al. Detection of colonic dysplasia in vivo using a targeted heptapeptide and confocal microendoscopy. Nat Med 2008;14(4):456; with permission.)

of exogenous probes, such as protease-activated, antibodies, and peptides, as targeting agents requires additional regulatory oversight beyond that provided by the local IRB. Although topical application of a molecular probe in the digestive tract is much safer than intravenous application, there remains some risk of a local reaction. Furthermore, the possibility of systemic toxicity will depend on the absorption and internalization properties of the specific probe. An investigational new drug (IND) application should be submitted to the FDA before the beginning of the study.[50] The contents of this application include an introductory statement, general investigational plan, study protocol, chemistry manufacturing and control (CMC) data, pharmacology and toxicology information, and any previous human experience. The introductory statement and general investigational plan provide a brief discussion of the study aims with sufficient background so that the FDA can understand the scope of the developmental plan and anticipate the future needs of the sponsor. The study protocol provides details about how clinical validation is to be performed, and includes the number of subjects, inclusion and exclusion criteria, dosing, monitoring (blood tests and survey), and stopping rules. The protocol for a Phase 1 study, with the primary goal of demonstrating safety, has flexibility to allow the sponsor to learn about probe function in vivo so that refinements can be made. The CMC provides details about the proper identification, quality, purity, stability, and concentration of the investigational probe, and the pharmacology section describes the probe's mechanism of action and provides information about its absorption, distribution, metabolism, and excretion. In addition, an animal toxicology study, typically performed on rats, is needed to support the safety of the molecular probe before introduction in human subjects. Finally, data from previous human experience can be provided if it exists.

SUMMARY AND FUTURE DIRECTIONS

In summary, several promising intracellular and cell surface targets expressed by the mucosa of the digestive tract have been identified that can reveal evidence of neoplastic transformation on endoscopic imaging. Exogenous probes are needed to interact with these targets, and novel fluorescence instruments, including wide-area endoscopy and confocal microscopy, are required for detection. Several classes of probes discussed in this text include protease-activated, antibody, and peptide probes. In addition, probes based on nanoparticle, aptamer, and small molecule platforms are also under development for this purpose. This novel, integrated imaging strategy promises to play an increasingly important role in the future management of patients who have an increased likelihood of developing cancer, including risk stratification, early detection, therapeutic monitoring, and evaluation of recurrence. The use of targeted imaging reveals functional information about the mucosa based on patterns of molecular expression, and in combination with the architectural features provided by conventional, reflected white light images, physicians will soon have a powerful new tool for diagnosing and treating patients with diseases of the digestive tract, including Barrett's esophagus, atrophic gastritis, and ulcerative colitis. To achieve these aims, more progress is needed in the development of molecular probes with high specificity, including improvement in target-to-background ratio, enhancement in delivery efficiency, and characterization of toxicity profiles. A greater understanding of the significance and timing of the overexpressed targets is needed. Improved endoscopic instruments that have multispectral detection capabilities and deeper tissue penetration imaging will be required. Finally, issues of interobserver variability, clinical efficacy, and cost effectiveness should be addressed with randomized, multicenter, controlled trials to validate and standardize the imaging methods. These promising techniques have great potential to improve detection sensitivity, increase surveillance efficiency, and ultimately achieve better patient outcomes for management of cancer in the digestive tract.

REFERENCES

1. Sivak MV. Gastrointestinal endoscopy: past and future. Gut 2006;55(8):1061–4.
2. Kumar V, Fausto N, Abbas A. Robbins & Cotran pathologic basis of disease. 7th edition. Philadelphia: WB Saunders Company; 2004.
3. Levine DS, Haggitt RC, Blount PL, et al. An endoscopic biopsy protocol can differentiate high-grade dysplasia from early adenocarcinoma in Barrett's esophagus. Gastroenterology 1993;105(1):40–50.
4. Jess T, Loftus EV Jr, Velayos FS, et al. Risk of intestinal cancer in inflammatory bowel disease: a population-based study from Olmsted County, Minnesota. Gastroenterology 2006;130(4):1039–46.
5. Vogelstein B, Kinzler KW. Cancer genes and the pathways they control. Nat Med 2004;10(8):789–99.
6. Serafini AN, Klein JL, Wolff BG, et al. Radioimmunoscintigraphy of recurrent, metastatic, or occult colorectal cancer with technetium 99m-labeled totally human

monoclonal antibody 88BV59: results of pivotal, phase III multicenter studies. J Clin Oncol 1998;16(5):1777–87.
7. Willkomm P, Bender H, Bangard M, et al. FDG PET and immunoscintigraphy with 99mTc-labeled antibody fragments for detection of the recurrence of colorectal carcinoma. J Nucl Med 2000;41(10):1657–63.
8. Weissleder R, Tung CH, Mahmood U, et al. In vivo imaging of tumors with protease-activated near-infrared fluorescent probes. Nat Biotechnol 1999;17(4): 375–8.
9. Tung CH, Mahmood U, Bredow S, et al. In vivo imaging of proteolytic enzyme activity using a novel molecular reporter. Cancer Res 2000;60(17):4953–8.
10. Bremer C, Bredow S, Mahmood U, et al. Optical imaging of matrix metalloproteinase-2 activity in tumors: feasibility study in a mouse model. Radiology 2001; 221(2):523–9.
11. Kang HW, Torres D, Wald L, et al. Targeted imaging of human endothelial-specific marker in a model of adoptive cell transfer. Lab Invest 2006;86(6):599–609.
12. Laxman B, Hall DE, Bhojani MS, et al. Noninvasive real-time imaging of apoptosis. Proc Natl Acad Sci U S A 2002;99(26):16551–5.
13. Messerli SM, Prabhakar S, Tang Y, et al. A novel method for imaging apoptosis using a caspase-1 near-infrared fluorescent probe. Neoplasia 2004;6(2): 95–105.
14. Maley CC, Galipeau PC, Finley JC, et al. Genetic clonal diversity predicts progression to esophageal adenocarcinoma. Nat Genet 2006;38(4):468–73.
15. Giacomini CP, Leung SY, Chen X, et al. A gene expression signature of genetic instability in colon cancer. Cancer Res 2005;65(20):9200–5.
16. Fitzgerald RC. Molecular basis of Barrett's oesophagus and oesophageal adenocarcinoma. Gut 2006;55(12):1810–20.
17. Syngal S, Clarke G, Bandipalliam P. Potential roles of genetic biomarkers in colorectal cancer chemoprevention. J Cell Biochem Suppl 2000;34:28–34.
18. Kruszewski WJ, Rzepko R, Wojtacki J, et al. Overexpression of cathepsin B correlates with angiogenesis in colon adenocarcinoma. Neoplasma 2004; 51(1):38–43.
19. McKerrow JH, Bhargava V, Hansell E, et al. A functional proteomics screen of proteases in colorectal carcinoma. Mol Med 2000;6(5):450–60.
20. Kioi M, Yamamoto K, Higashi S, et al. Matrilysin (MMP-7) induces homotypic adhesion of human colon cancer cells and enhances their metastatic potential in nude mouse model. Oncogene 2003;22(54):8662–70.
21. Tanioka Y, Yoshida T, Yagawa T, et al. Matrix metalloproteinase-7 and matrix metalloproteinase-9 are associated with unfavourable prognosis in superficial oesophageal cancer. Br J Cancer 2003;89(11):2116–21.
22. Folli S, Wagnières G, Pèlegrin A, et al. Immunophotodiagnosis of colon carcinomas in patients injected with fluoresceinated chimeric antibodies against carcinoembryonic antigen. Proc Natl Acad Sci U S A 1992;89(17):7973–7.
23. Ito S, Muguruma N, Kusaka Y, et al. Detection of human gastric cancer in resected specimens using a novel infrared fluorescent anti-human carcinoembryonic antigen antibody with an infrared fluorescence endoscope in vitro. Endoscopy 2001;33(10):849–53.
24. Sagara M, Yonezawa S, Nagata K, et al. Expression of mucin 1 (MUC1) in esophageal squamous-cell carcinoma: its relationship with prognosis. Int J Cancer 1999;84(3):251–7.

25. Utsunomiya T, Yonezawa S, Sakamoto H, et al. Expression of MUC1 and MUC2 mucins in gastric carcinomas: its relationship with the prognosis of the patients. Clin Cancer Res 1998;4(11):2605–14.
26. Schechter AL, Hung MC, Vaidyanathan L, et al. The neu gene: an erbB-homologous gene distinct from and unlinked to the gene encoding the EGF receptor. Science 1985;229(4717):976–8.
27. Yu D, Hung MC. Overexpression of ErbB2 in cancer and ErbB2-targeting strategies. Oncogene 2000;19(53):6115–21.
28. Ortega P, Morán A, de Juan C, et al. Differential Wnt pathway gene expression and E-cadherin truncation in sporadic colorectal cancers with and without microsatellite instability. Clin Cancer Res 2008;14(4):995–1001.
29. Marten K, Bremer C, Khazaie K, et al. Detection of dysplastic intestinal adenomas using enzyme-sensing molecular beacons in mice. Gastroenterology 2002; 122(2):406–14.
30. Alencar H, Funovics MA, Figueiredo J, et al. Colonic adenocarcinomas: near-infrared microcatheter imaging of smart probes for early detection–study in mice. Radiology 2007;244(1):232–8.
31. Kuusela P, Jalanko H, Roberts P, et al. Comparison of CA 19-9 and carcinoembryonic antigen (CEA) levels in the serum of patients with colorectal diseases. Br J Cancer 1984;49(2):135–9.
32. Reichelt U, Duesedau P, Tsourlakis MCh, et al. Frequent homogeneous HER-2 amplification in primary and metastatic adenocarcinoma of the esophagus. Mod Pathol 2007;20(1):120–9.
33. Pegram MD, Reese DM. Combined biological therapy of breast cancer using monoclonal antibodies directed against HER2/neu protein and vascular endothelial growth factor. Semin Oncol 2002;29(3 Suppl 11):29–37.
34. Emlet DR, Brown KA, Kociban DL, et al. Response to trastuzumab, erlotinib, and bevacizumab, alone and in combination, is correlated with the level of human epidermal growth factor receptor-2 expression in human breast cancer cell lines. Mol Cancer Ther 2007;6(10):2664–74.
35. Rauser S, Weis R, Braselmann H, et al. Significance of HER2 low-level copy gain in Barrett's cancer: implications for fluorescence in situ hybridization testing in tissues. Clin Cancer Res 2007;13(17):5115–23.
36. Arteaga CL, O'Neill A, Moulder SL, et al. A phase I-II study of combined blockade of the ErbB receptor network with trastuzumab and gefitinib in patients with HER2 (ErbB2)-overexpressing metastatic breast cancer. Clin Cancer Res 2008;14(19): 6277–83.
37. Medina PJ, Goodin S. Lapatinib: a dual inhibitor of human epidermal growth factor receptor tyrosine kinases. Clin Ther 2008;30(8):1426–47.
38. Funovics M, Weissleder R, Tung CH. Protease sensors for bioimaging. Anal Bioanal Chem 2003;377(6):956–63.
39. Available at: http://www.visenmedical.com. Accessed March 30, 2009.
40. Keller R, Winde G, Terpe HJ, et al. Fluorescence endoscopy using a fluorescein-labeled monoclonal antibody against carcinoembryonic antigen in patients with colorectal carcinoma and adenoma. Endoscopy 2002;34(10):801–7.
41. Bando T, Muguruma N, Ito S, et al. Basic studies on a labeled anti-mucin antibody detectable by infrared-fluorescence endoscopy. J Gastroenterol 2002;37(4): 260–9.
42. Kelly K, Alencar H, Funovics M, et al. Detection of invasive colon cancer using a novel, targeted, library-derived fluorescent peptide. Cancer Res 2004;64(17): 6247–51.

43. Lu S, Wang TD. In vivo cancer biomarkers of esophageal neoplasia. Cancer Biomark 2008;4(6):341–50.
44. Hsiung PL, Hardy J, Friedland S, et al. Detection of colonic dysplasia in vivo using a targeted heptapeptide and confocal microendoscopy. Nat Med 2008;14(4):454–8.
45. Ito S, Muguruma N, Kimura T, et al. Principle and clinical usefulness of the infrared fluorescence endoscopy. J Med Invest 2006;53(1–2):1–8.
46. Uedo N, Higashino K, Ishihara R, et al. Diagnosis of colonic adenomas by new autofluorescence imaging system: a pilot study. Digestive Endoscopy 2007;19(S1):S134–8.
47. Pawley J, editor. Handbook of biological confocal microscopy. 3rd edition. New York: Plenum; 1996.
48. Kiesslich R, Burg J, Vieth M, et al. Confocal laser endoscopy for diagnosing intraepithelial neoplasias and colorectal cancer in vivo. Gastroenterology 2004;127(3):706–13.
49. Wang TD, Friedland S, Sahbaie P, et al. Functional imaging of colonic mucosa with a fibered confocal microscope for real-time in vivo pathology. Clin Gastroenterol Hepatol 2007;5(11):1300–5.
50. US Food and Drug Administration. Available at: http://www.fda.gov/CDER. Accessed March 30, 2009.

New Endoscopic and Cytologic Tools for Cancer Surveillance in the Digestive Tract

Eric J. Seibel, PhD[a,*], Teresa A. Brentnall, MD[b], Jason A. Dominitz, MD, MHS[c,d]

KEYWORDS

• Endoscope • Biopsy • Image-guided intervention
• Three-dimensional cytology • Cancer surveillance

Cancer surveillance is an increasing part of everyday practice in gastrointestinal (GI) endoscopy due to the identification of high-risk groups from genetic and biomarker testing, genealogic and epidemiologic studies, and the increasing number of cancer survivors. For colorectal cancer, Winawer and colleagues[1] report that there is growing demand for colonoscopy resources for postpolypectomy surveillance as well as screening. For example, there is a need to shift emphasis from the diagnosis of symptomatic pancreatic cancer to screening (and surveillance) of asymptomatic individuals at high risk.[2] Surveillance strategies developed for patients with hereditary pancreatic cancer can be used as a model for other high-risk groups.[3] Thus, a major goal for the endoscopist and biomedical engineer is to move toward more preemptive and preventative procedures that will ultimately reduce GI cancer mortality rates.[4]

The challenge for the next generation of endoscopic imaging is to improve the efficiency, sensitivity, and accuracy of disease detection and site selection for biopsy and cell sampling. Because many of the tissue and cellular features of precancer and early

Funding: As principal investigator, Eric Seibel received funding in support of this project from the following sources: NIH/NCI (CA094303), NSF (CBET-0809070), PENTAX (HOYA Corp., Tokyo, Japan), and VisionGate Inc., (Gig Harbor, WA). Jason Dominitz is supported by an ASGE Career Development Award and NIH/NCI grant CA128231.

[a] Department of Mechanical Engineering, Adjunct Bioengineering, Human Photonics Laboratory, University of Washington, Box 352600, Seattle, WA 98195, USA

[b] Department of Medicine, University of Washington, 1959 NE Pacific Street, Box 356424, Seattle, WA 98195, USA

[c] Department of Medicine, Division of Gastroenterology, University of Washington School of Medicine, Seattle, WA 98195, USA

[d] Northwest Hepatitis C Resource Center, VA Puget Sound Health Care System, 1660 S. Columbian Way (111-Gastro), Seattle, WA 98108, USA

* Corresponding author.

E-mail address: eseibel@u.washington.edu (E.J. Seibel).

Gastrointest Endoscopy Clin N Am 19 (2009) 299–307
doi:10.1016/j.giec.2009.02.002
giendo.theclinics.com

stage cancers are not visible using standard endoscopic tools, new technologies will need to be developed. These new endoscopic tools should be developed and tested not just for the main GI tract but also for the smaller pancreatic and biliary ducts. In this technology report on the state of ultrathin and flexible laser scanning endoscopy, new endoscopic and cytologic tools are introduced for cost-effective cancer surveillance of the esophagus as well as the smaller pancreaticobiliary ducts reached by endoscopic retrograde cholangiopancreatography (ERCP). These proposed tools are expected to be widely applicable to clinical practice for cancer screening and surveillance within the fields of gynecology, pulmonology, and urology, in addition to gastroenterology.

At the University of Washington, a new endoscopic imaging technology has been developed for two GI applications: the tethered-capsule endoscope (TCE) for esophageal imaging and the scanning fiber endoscope (SFE) for small duct imaging. Both endoscopes produce images in the same, but unique way.[5,6] The distal tip of a single illumination optical fiber is scanned in a spiral pattern. Narrow bands of red, green, and blue (RGB) laser light are scanned over the tissue at wide field of view (100°). The collected light from this flying-spot scan is detected in time series, one pixel at a time, from the light collected by a ring of optical fibers that surround the micro-optical scanner. Unlike video chip endoscopes, the number of pixels within an image is not determined by the number of camera sensor elements or collection optical fibers. The number of pixels in the TCE and SFE images is a user-controlled feature ultimately limited by optical performance of the lens system. Current TCE and SFE prototypes operate at 30 Hz for 500-line color images or 15 Hz for 1,000-line color images. The size of the SFE is currently 1.2 mm in overall diameter with a rigid tip length of less than 10 mm (**Fig. 1**). The capsule size of the TCE is 18 mm in length and 6.4 mm in overall diameter, which is a standard size for over-the-counter pills (**Fig. 2**), whereas the soft supple tether is 1.4 mm in diameter. The capsule design was implemented to facilitate swallowing. As the SFE and TCE probes are composed of low-cost components, these probes could be manufactured at high volume for single use, although reprocessing is currently under investigation.

PROPOSED ESOPHAGEAL SURVEILLANCE USING TCE WITH IMAGE CONTRAST ENHANCEMENT

Barrett's esophagus is a precancerous change in the esophagus associated with gastroesophageal reflux. Screening and surveillance for Barrett's esophagus is performed to look for dysplasia, the histologic change that precedes cancer. The determination of dysplasia is difficult with conventional endoscopic technology because dysplastic tissue is rarely visible.[7] Surface mucosal treatments of chomoendoscopy have been developed to increase the image contrast of dysplastic mucosal patterns with some successes,[8] but an accessory channel is required for topical application of dye. Instead of modifying the tissue, the endoscope can be modified for higher intensity blue light illumination to detect the surface mucosal thickening that is associated with neoplasia in patients with Barrett's esophagus.[9] Alternatively, the spectral content of the endoscopic illumination can be varied to increase contrast of mucosal and vascular patterns,[10] but magnification can be a requirement to achieve detection rate advantages over white-light imaging.[11]

Magnification and enhanced spectral imaging (ESI) are standard imaging features of the tethered-capsule endoscope, which uses narrow laser bands for illumination. The unique aspect of the TCE is that the ESI image contrast enhancement can be applied in real time with a user-controlled switch or by postprocessing the digitally stored color video images. In **Figs. 3** and **4**, both types of ESI enhancements are shown from single

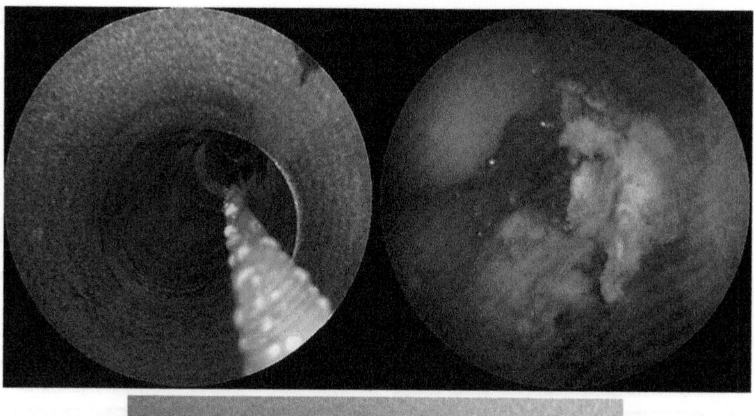

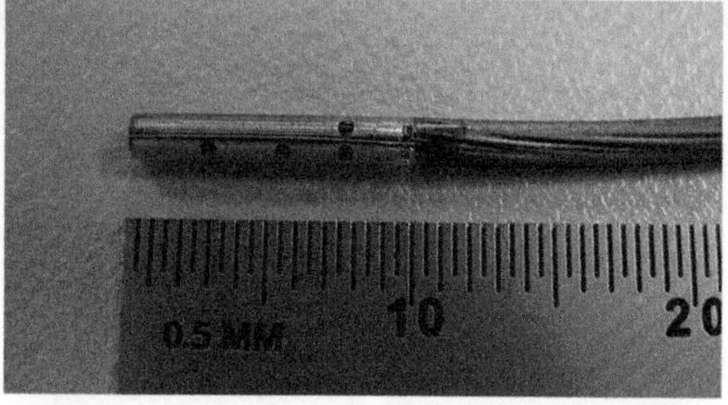

Fig. 1. SFE images during in vivo imaging in a pig bile duct using ERCP. (*Top left*) The 4.2-mm working channel and guidewire; (*top right*) an SFE image frame. (*Lower image*) An SFE probe with 9-mm rigid tip length and 1.2-mm overall diameter. (*Reprinted from* Seibel EJ, Melville CD, Johnston RS, et al. Bile duct imaging with ultrathin laser scanning catheterscope in a swine model. Gastrointest Endosc 2008;67(5):AB133–4; with permission.)

500-line video frames acquired during 30-Hz operation (no image averaging). In **Fig. 3**, a TCE image of normal contrast can be compared with TCE video frames with the ESI feature taken from approximately the same region of the human inner cheek at different magnifications and different locations. In **Fig. 4**, a TCE image taken at the

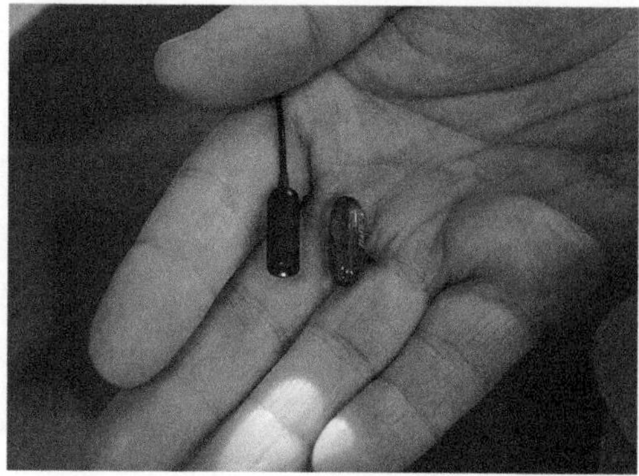

Fig. 2. The TCE probe and an ibuprofen gel capsule (Advil, Wyeth) for size comparison. (*Courtesy of* Rob Watters, Seattle, WA.)

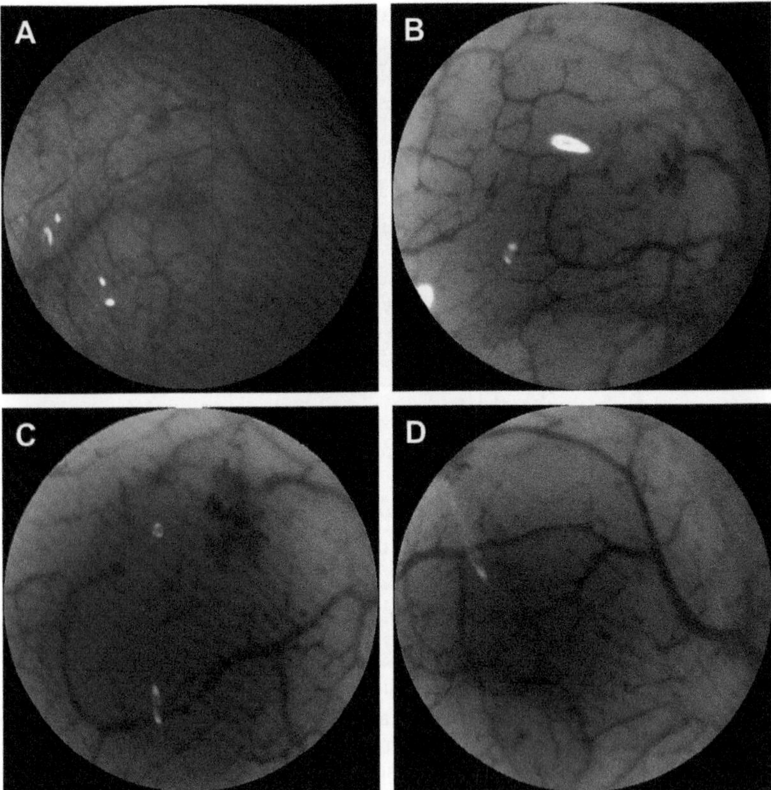

Fig. 3. TCE images showing a video frame in normal operation (*A*) and subsequent video frames captured with the enhanced spectral imaging (ESI) feature applied (*B*). TCE with ESI is demonstrated with increased magnification within the previous field of view (*C*), and in a new region of the human cheek (*D*).

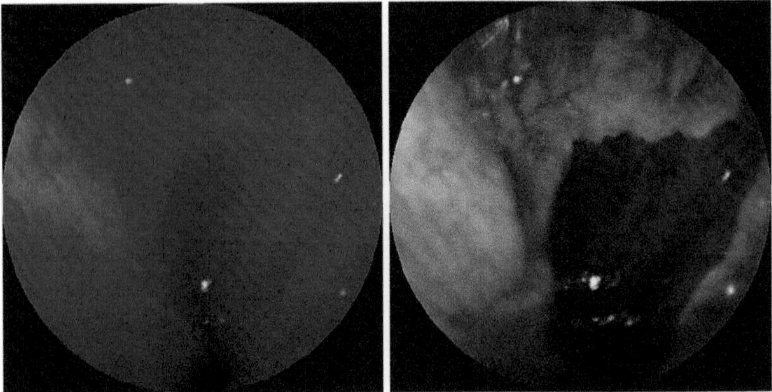

Fig. 4. TCE video frame acquired and digitally stored during examination of the lower esophagus in human subjects. Normal TCE contrast is displayed on the left, and the same TCE video frame is postprocessed with enhanced spectral imaging (*right*).

lower human esophagus during normal operation has been digitally stored and ESI contrast has been postprocessed for comparison. Currently, TCE magnification is limited to approximately 130× real magnification, corresponding to resolution of features measuring 15 microns. The light exposure of the combined RGB laser illumination is equivalent to the standard illumination levels from white-light endoscopy, roughly the same as using three continuously scanned laser pointers.

A tethered capsule is not considered a new device for gastroenterology, as they have been used for more than 30 years for obtaining tissue biopsies from the small intestine of children and adults.[12,13] Often these biopsies from tethered capsules provide equivalent histologic results to endoscopy, although the endoscopic procedure is considered advantageous due to a faster procedure, direct visualization of the bowel, and collection of many biopsy samples.[14] The TCE with high-quality video now provides direct visualization and a fast procedure time for imaging the lower esophagus perorally, without the use of any anesthetic or sedation. Recently, an air channel was added to the TCE tether and comfortably swallowed, allowing the user to control the distention of the esophagus and to remove bubbles.[15] Thus, with the existence of a micro-optical scanner for video-rate imaging and a side channel, the ability to add image-guided biopsy and simple interventions may be forthcoming.

PROPOSED SMALL DUCT SURVEILLANCE USING SFE AS A CATHETERSCOPE

The SFE provides excellent image quality from 1-mm diameter catheter-style endoscopes, which are analogous to a "guidewire with eyes." In the standard ERCP procedure, the SFE with less than 10-mm rigid tip length can be introduced into either the biliary or pancreatic duct through the working channel of a side-viewing therapeutic duodenoscope (see **Fig. 1**[16]). However, a steerable SFE would be preferable to navigate through the pancreatobiliary ducts and to reduce the forces applied to the walls of the ducts. Similar to a cardiovascular catheter, the capability for tip deflection can be added without increasing the size of the rigid tip and flexible shaft. Replacing the central wire within a cardiovascular catheter with the single illumination optical fiber of the SFE as the central compression element allows tip deflection by pulling on a pair of peripheral wires or the optical fibers used for light collection (**Fig. 5**). The new endoscopic tool is a catheterscope with 4-way tip bending or steerable "guidewire with eyes." Along this guidewire, cannula-style tools (brush, needle/tube, forceps) can be introduced into small ducts for image-guided interventions. Previously, a multimodal optical fiber was incorporated into the forceps for point spectroscopic measurements of GI cancers before biopsy.[17] In our case, the annular gap that surrounds the proposed 1-mm SFE can be used for extracting cells and fluid samples from ducts smaller than 2 mm in diameter using a brush (**Fig. 6**). Tissue core samples and aspirants may be extracted using a needle with SFE as the central plunger. Custom 2-mm diameter mini-pancreatoscopes are preferred over larger endoscopes as sphincterotomy is not required with the smaller scope.[18] Future clinical testing will be necessary to determine if small duct surveillance could be performed in a modified ERCP procedure that may not require fluoroscopy.

THREE-DIMENSIONAL CYTOLOGY OF CELL SAMPLES FROM PROPOSED SFE CANNULA TOOLS

Although biomarker detection of disease within the GI tract is an ultimate goal, cell/tissue removal is required for diagnosis. Smaller cellular samples are less invasive, but without tissue architecture, standard cytology has been proved to lack sensitivity. At the University of Washington a new optical microscope that can provide three-dimensional images for cytologic analysis has been codeveloped with VisionGate

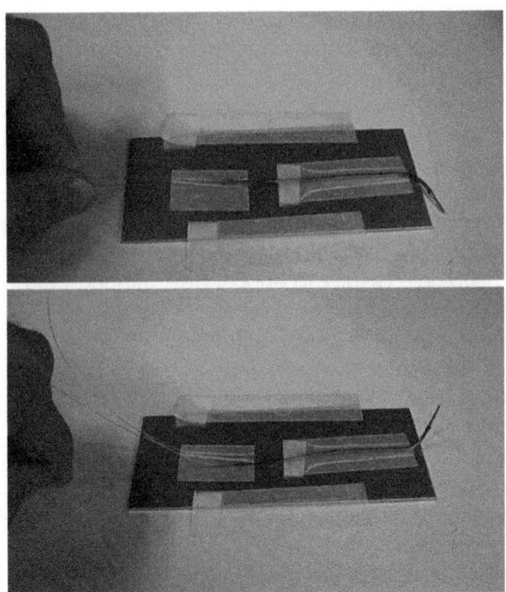

Fig. 5. Tip bending in a 1.5-mm diameter SFE probe during manufacture.

Inc. (Gig Harbor, Washington).[19] Fixed hematoxylin-stained cells are imaged in a transmission-like standard cytologic examination. However, these cells are then rotated and re-imaged from 250 perspectives within 360° to produce three-dimensional images of submicrometer isometric resolution. Reconstructed three-dimensional images are generated in the same manner as three-dimensional radiographic images are generated using computed tomography (CT). Representative Cell-CT images of a cultured pancreatic cancer cell (PaTu1) are shown in grayscale in a series of perspectives, along with two images with pseudocolor thresholds set to highlight the nuclear membrane and internal nuclear chromatin-dense structures (**Fig. 7**). In a controlled comparison test on the same human cultured cells (A549 lung adenocarcinoma cells and small airway epithelial cells), the use of a classifier using

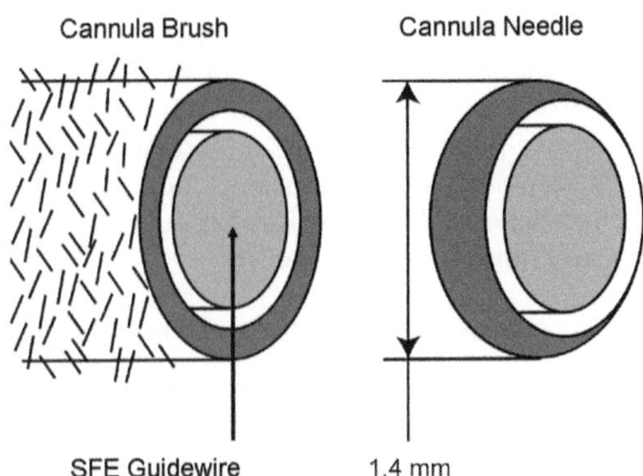

Fig. 6. Cannula-style tools of brush and needle depicted around a future 1-mm SFE probe as a steerable guidewire with eyes.

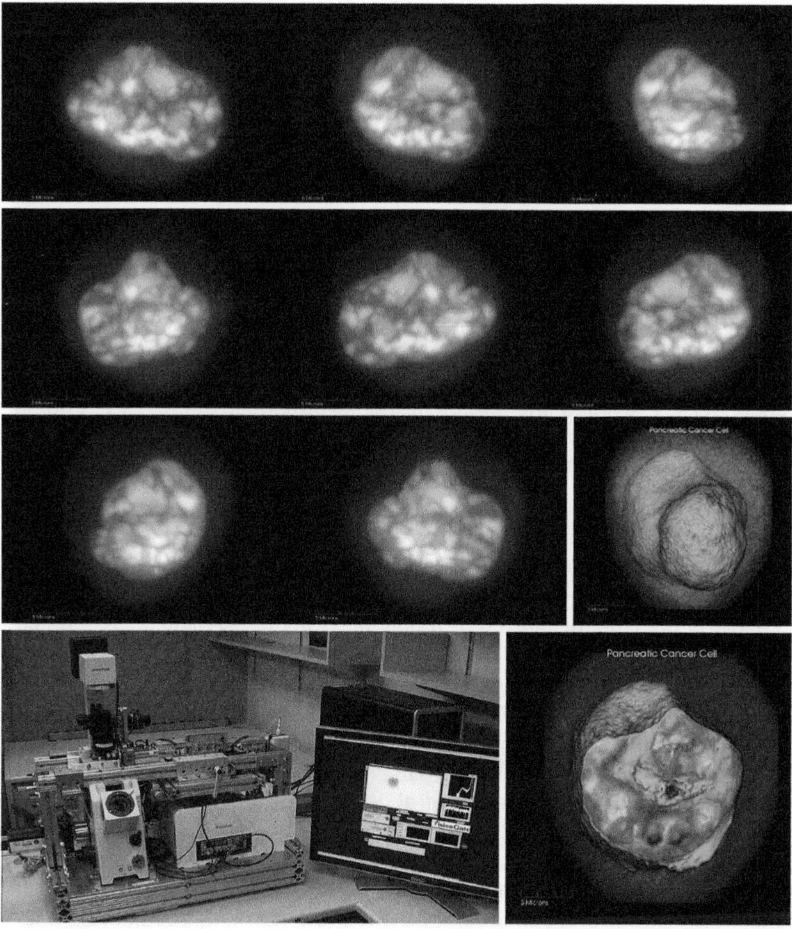

Fig. 7. Cell-CT instrument and transmission images of human pancreatic cancer cell (PaTu1, alcohol-fixed, hematoxylin-stained) shown in grayscale in series of different rotational perspectives. The same cell is visualized using Volview software with thresholding set to opacify the irregular nuclear envelope (*blue*) and highlight chromatin-dense bodies within a slice of nucleus (*red*).

three-dimensional cytologic features versus standard cytology reduced the false negative rate by threefold at the same 96% specificity.[20] The improved sensitivity of three-dimensional cytologic imaging and analysis in this preliminary study provides an incentive for the long-term success of small duct surveillance using less invasive microbiopsy tools.

SUMMARY

Scanning fiber endoscope technology is demonstrated as a platform technology on which future clinical protocols will be developed for cancer surveillance. In the esophagus, the tethered-capsule endoscope with enhanced spectral imaging can be used without sedation, which lowers the cost and reduces barriers for esophageal cancer screening and surveillance. In the pancreatic and biliary ducts, SFE technology with cannula tools can provide high-quality image guidance for biopsy, and is smaller in size and has greater flexibility than current endoscope technology. Finally, the anticipated increase in sensitivity from three-dimensional cytologic analysis of cell samples from these small ducts should provide the necessary clinical tools required for a successful endoscopic cancer surveillance program for the pancreas and bile ducts.

ACKNOWLEDGMENTS

Engineering of the new endoscopic tools was provided by Dave Melville, Rich Johnston, and Cameron Lee from the Human Photonics Laboratory. The new cytologic instrument and three-dimensional visualization was engineered by Michael Meyer, Richard Rahn, Florence Patten, Julia Yu, Mark Fauver, Thomas Neumann, and Alan C. Nelson of VisionGate Inc., Gig Harbor, WA. Cell-CT is a trademark registered by Visiongate Inc. Technical support was received by David Crispin on the cultured pancreatic cancer cells. The first author gratefully thanks attendees of the ASGE course, The Next Generation in Endoscopic Imaging, Dallas, TX, who provided information on tethered-capsule devices for small bowel biopsy.

REFERENCES

1. Winawer SJ, Zauber AG, Fletcher RH, et al. Guidelines for colonoscopy surveillance after polypectomy: a consensus update by the Multi-Society Task Force on Colorectal Cancer and the American Cancer Society. Gastroenterology 2006;130(6):1872–85.
2. Canto MI. Screening and surveillance approaches in familial pancreatic cancer. Gastrointest Endosc Clin N Am 2008;18(3):535–53.
3. Brentnall TA. Management strategies for patients with hereditary pancreatic cancer. Curr Treat Options Oncol 2005;6(5):437–45.
4. Kelloff GJ, Sullivan DC, Baker H, et al. Workshop on imaging science development for cancer prevention and preemption. Cancer Biomark 2007;3(1):1–33.
5. Seibel EJ, Carroll R, Dominitz JA, et al. Tethered capsule endoscopy, a low-cost and high-performance alternative technology for the screening of esophageal cancer and Barrett's esophagus. IEEE Trans Biomed Eng 2008;55(3):1032–42.
6. Seibel EJ, Brown CM, Dominitz JA, et al. Scanning single fiber endoscopy: a new platform technology for integrated laser imaging, diagnosis, and future therapies. Gastrointest Endosc Clin N Am 2008;18:467–78.
7. Wilson BC. Detection and treatment of dysplasia in Barrett's esophagus: a pivotal challenge in translating biophotonics from bench to bedside. J Biomed Opt 2007;12(5):051401-1-22.
8. ASGE Technology Committee. Technology status evaluation report: chromoendoscopy. Gastrointest Endosc 2007;66(4):639–49.
9. Kara MA, Peters FP, ten Kate FJW, et al. Endoscopic video autofluorescence imaging may improve the detection of early neoplasia in patients with Barrett's esophagus. Gastrointest Endosc 2005;61(6):679–85.
10. Sharma P, Bansal A, Mathur S, et al. The utility of a novel narrow band imaging endoscopy system in patients with Barrett's esophagus. Gastrointest Endosc 2006;64(2):167–239.
11. Friedland S. Narrow band imaging of the bile duct. Gastrointest Endosc 2007;66(4):737–8.
12. Dickey W, Porter KG. Perendoscopic Watson capsule biopsy of the jejunum: a simple, effective, safe method which does not require fluoroscopy. Gastrointest Endosc 1995;41(1):81–2.

13. Branski D, Faber J, Freier S, et al. Histologic evaluation of endoscopic versus suction biopsies of small intestinal mucosae in children with and without celiac disease. J Pediatr Gastroenterol Nutr 1998;27(1):6–11.
14. Gottrand F, Michaud L, Guimber D, et al. Comparison of fiberendoscopy and suction capsule for small intestinal biopsy in children with and without celiac disease. J Pediatr Gastroenterol Nutr 1999;28(3):353.
15. Seibel EJ, Melville CD, Lung JKC, et al. Swallowable capsule with air channel for improved image-guided cancer detection in the esophagus, Medical Imaging 2009: Visualization, Image-guided Procedures, and Modeling, Proc SPIE 2009;7261:72611C-1-7.
16. Seibel EJ, Melville CD, Johnston RS, et al. Bile duct imaging with ultrathin laser scanning catheterscope in a swine model. Gastrointest Endosc 2008;67(5): AB133–4.
17. Wong Kee Song L-M, Marcon NE. Fluorescence and Raman spectroscopy. Gastrointest Endosc Clin N Am 2003;13:279–96.
18. Kodama T, Tatsumi Y, Sato H, et al. Initial experience with a new peroral electronic pancreatoscope with an accessory channel. Gastrointest Endosc 2004;59(7): 895–900.
19. Fauver M, Seibel EJ, Rahn JR, et al. Three-dimensional imaging of single isolated cell nuclei using optical projection tomography. Opt Express 2005;13(11): 4210–23.
20. Meyer MG, Fauver M, Rahn JR, et al. Automated cellular analysis in 2D and 3D: a comparative study. Pattern Recognit 2009;42(1):141–6.

Index

Note: Page numbers of article titles are in **boldface** type.

Gastrointest Endoscopy Clin N Am 19 (2009) 309–314
doi:10.1016/S1052-5157(09)00053-1 giendo.theclinics.com
1052-5157/09/$ – see front matter

H

I

L

M

O

P

R

S

T